MEDICAL TERMINOLOGY CROSSWORDS

volume 1 | Easy Level

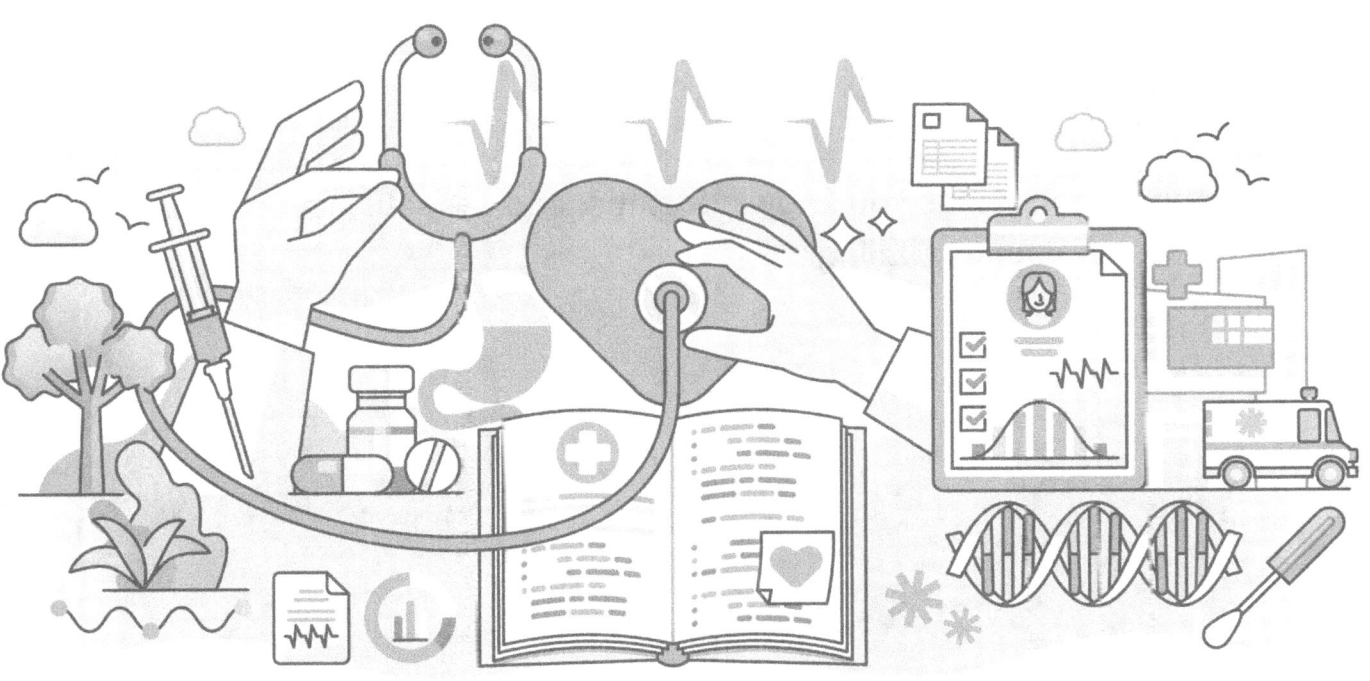

Emmy Dittman

Welcome to Medical Terminology Crosswords!

This book is crafted for medical students, healthcare professionals, and anyone with a passion for medicine. Whether you're exploring medical specialties, clinical cases, or the latest innovations in healthcare, these crosswords will offer you a fun and enriching experience.

With 90 puzzles and more than 1,000 medical terms, this book provides hours of enjoyment while expanding your understanding of key medical concepts. Dive into each puzzle and discover the fascinating world of medicine in an engaging and interactive way.

We hope this book brings you knowledge, fun, and the satisfaction of solving each crossword. Happy puzzling!

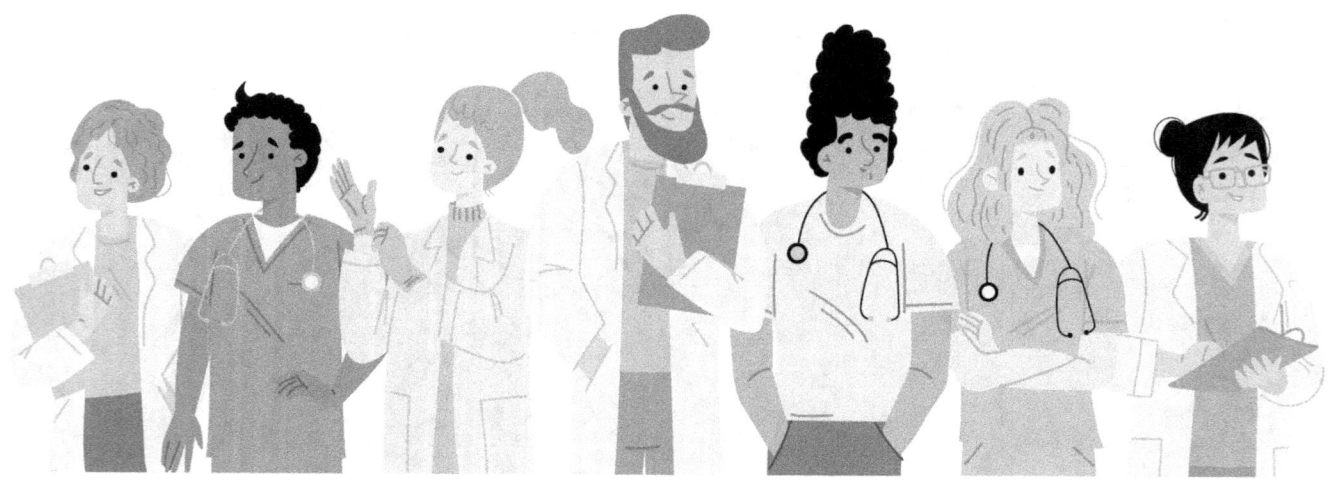

Table of CONTENTS

MEDICAL SPECIALTIES — PAGES

1. Cardiology — 06
2. Neurology — 07
3. Oncology — 08
4. Dermatology — 09
5. Orthopedics — 10
6. Gastroenterology — 11
7. Pulmonology — 12
8. Endocrinology — 13
9. Nephrology — 14
10. Rheumatology — 15
11. Ophthalmology — 16
12. Otolaryngology (ENT) — 17
13. Hematology — 18
14. Pediatrics — 19
15. Geriatrics — 20
16. Obstetrics And Gynecology (OB-GYN) — 21
17. Psychiatry — 22
18. Radiology — 23
19. Anesthesiology — 24
20. Urology — 25
21. Infectious Diseases — 26
22. Immunology — 27
23. Pathology — 28
24. Plastic Surgery — 29
25. Emergency Medicine — 30

MEDICAL GENERALITIES AND MISCELLANEOUS

26. Famous Medical Discoveries — 31
27. Nobel Prize In Medicine — 32
28. Ancient Medicine — 33
29. Medical Pioneers — 34
30. Men's Health — 35
31. Medical Devices — 36
32. Surgical Techniques — 37
33. Human Anatomy — 38
34. Environmental Health — 39
35. Nutrition And Dietetics — 40
36. Women's Health — 41

37	Alternative Medicine	42
38	Parasites	43
39	Exploring Toxicology	44
40	Biochemical Pathways	45
41	Medical Ethics	46
42	Pharmacology	47
43	Bacteriology	48
44	Emergency Prescriptions	49
45	Fungal Biology	50
46	Lab Diagnostics	51
47	Pediatric Pathologies	52
48	Virology Basics	53
49	Entomological Diseases	54
50	Famous Medical Journals	55

CLINICAL CASES

51	A Sweet But Dangerous Condition	56
52	The Silent Pressure Within	57
53	Breathless In The Night	58
54	A Breathless Battle	59
55	When The Heart's Pathways Are Blocked	60
56	A Sudden Loss Of Connection	61
57	A Joint Affair	62
58	A Slow Decline In Function	63
59	Bones Of Glass	64
60	The Memory Thief	65
61	The Shaky Path Forward	66
62	A Burning Question	67
63	The Unsettled Gut	68
64	A Liver's Silent Enemy	69
65	The Immune System's Hidden Battle	70
66	A Persistent Shadow In The Lungs	71
67	The Thin Red Line	72
68	A Gland's Wild Ride	73
69	A Mind In Turmoil	74
70	A Rash Decision	75
71	A Vein's Treacherous Path	76
72	The Silent Blood Thief	77
73	A Clouded Mind	78
74	The Hidden Uterine Battle	79
75	An Overflow Of Red	80

MEDICAL INNOVATIONS AND BREAKTHROUGHS

76 __ The Dawn Of Antibiotics _____ 81
77 __ The Birth Of Modern Surgery _____ 82
78 __ Supplements Uncovered _____ 83
79 __ Pioneering The Pacemaker _____ 84
80 __ A New Look Inside _____ 85
81 __ Vaccines That Changed The World _____ 86
82 __ Reviving Health With Ai _____ 87
83 __ Regenerative Revolution _____ 88
84 __ Innovation In Surgical Interventions _____ 89
85 __ Revolutionizing Cancer Care _____ 90
86 __ Innovations In Treating Neurological Disorders. _____ 91
87 __ Smart Implants _____ 92
88 __ Crispr Gene Editing _____ 93
89 __ Defenders Against Viruses _____ 94
90 __ Biologics : The Next Generation Of Medicine _____ 95

SOLUTIONS _____ 96

PUZZLE 01
CARDIOLOGY

Medical Specialties

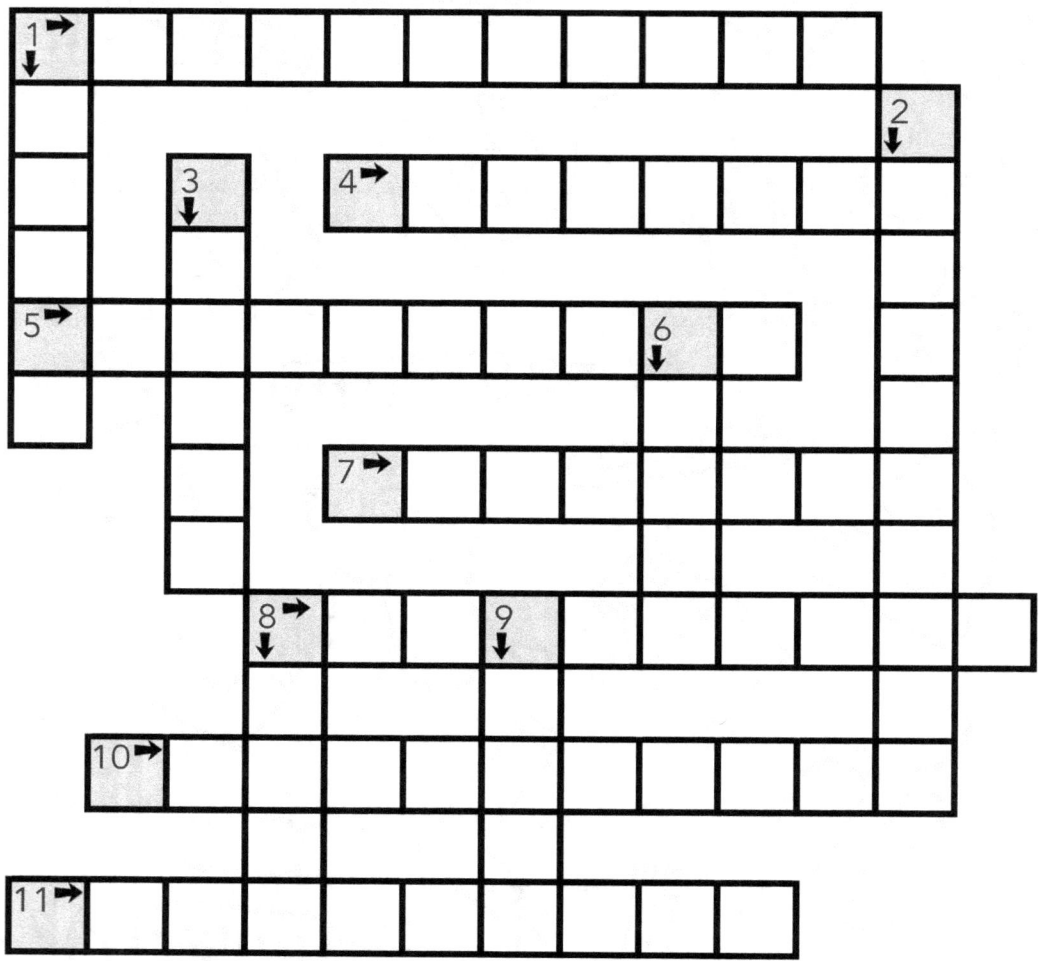

ACROSS

1. Medication that reduces heart rate and blood pressure.
4. Relating to blood vessels supplying the heart muscle.
5. Cardiovascular examination during controlled exercise.
7. Thin tube inserted into blood vessels or body cavities.
8. Irregular heartbeat or abnormal heart rhythm.
10. Protective membrane surrounding the heart.
11. Tissue death due to inadequate blood supply.

DOWN

1. Surgical rerouting of blood flow around blocked arteries.
2. Muscular tissue of the heart wall.
3. Upper chamber of the heart.
6. Expandable tube to keep arteries open.
8. Largest artery in the body.
9. Central blood-pumping organ.

Solution on page 96

PUZZLE 02
NEUROLOGY

Medical Specialties

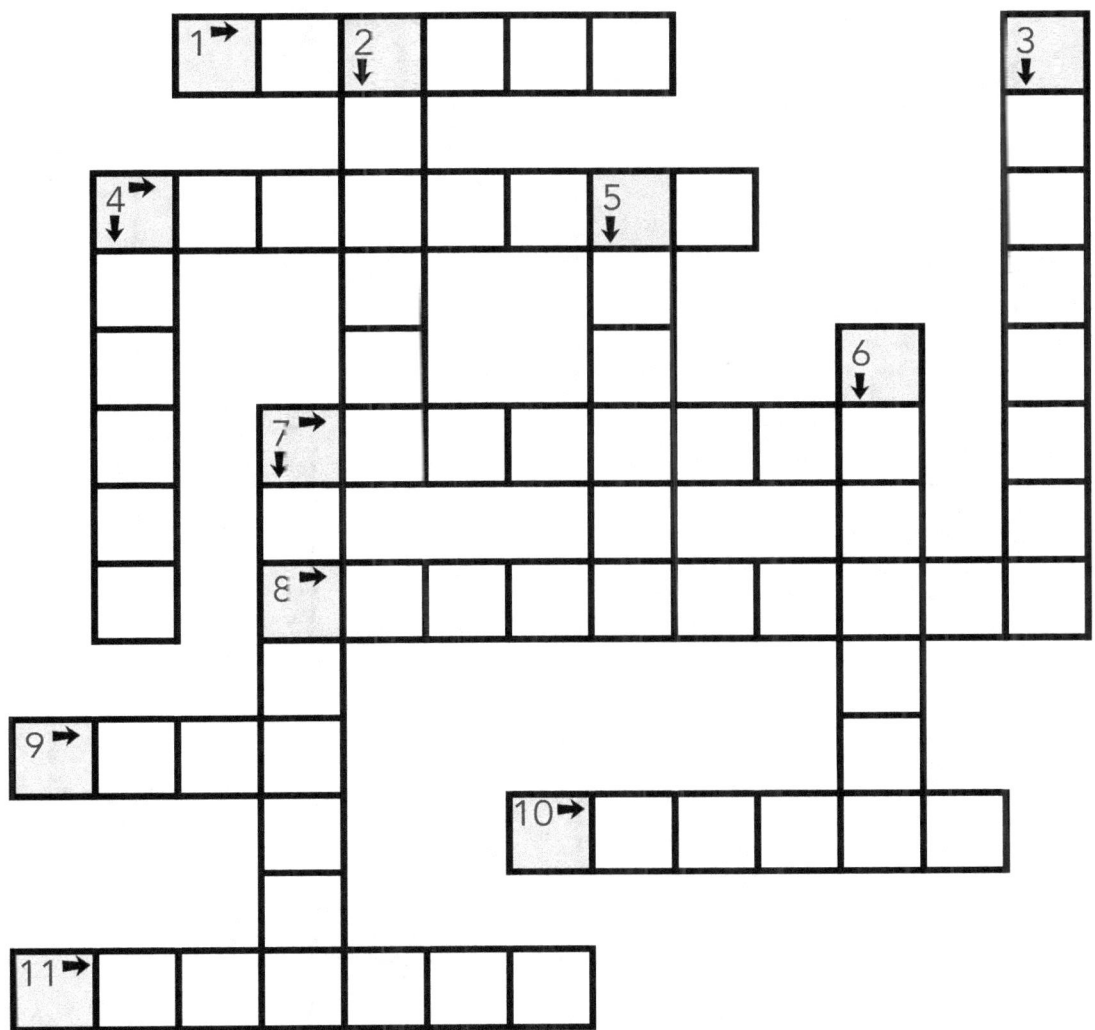

ACROSS
1. Cross-sectional imaging technique.
4. Severe recurring headache.
7. Branched neuronal extension.
8. Inflammation of brain membranes.
9. Nerve fiber conducting impulses.
10. Involuntary rhythmic movement.
11. Junction between neurons.

DOWN
2. Acute cerebrovascular event.
3. Sensory relay center.
4. Insulating nerve sheath.
5. Basic nerve cell unit.
6. Sensation of spinning.
7. Progressive cognitive decline.

Solution on page 96

PUZZLE 03
ONCOLOGY

Medical Specialties

ACROSS

1. Site of hematopoiesis.
8. Gene promoting tumor growth.
9. Reduction of cancer symptoms.
10. Connective tissue malignancy.
11. Abnormal mass of cells.

DOWN

2. Formation of new blood vessels.
3. Tending to invade and metastasize.
4. Imaging technique using radiotracers.
5. Blood cell cancer.
6. Cancer specialist physician.
7. Epithelial tissue cancer.

Solution on page 96

PUZZLE 04
DERMATOLOGY

Medical Specialties

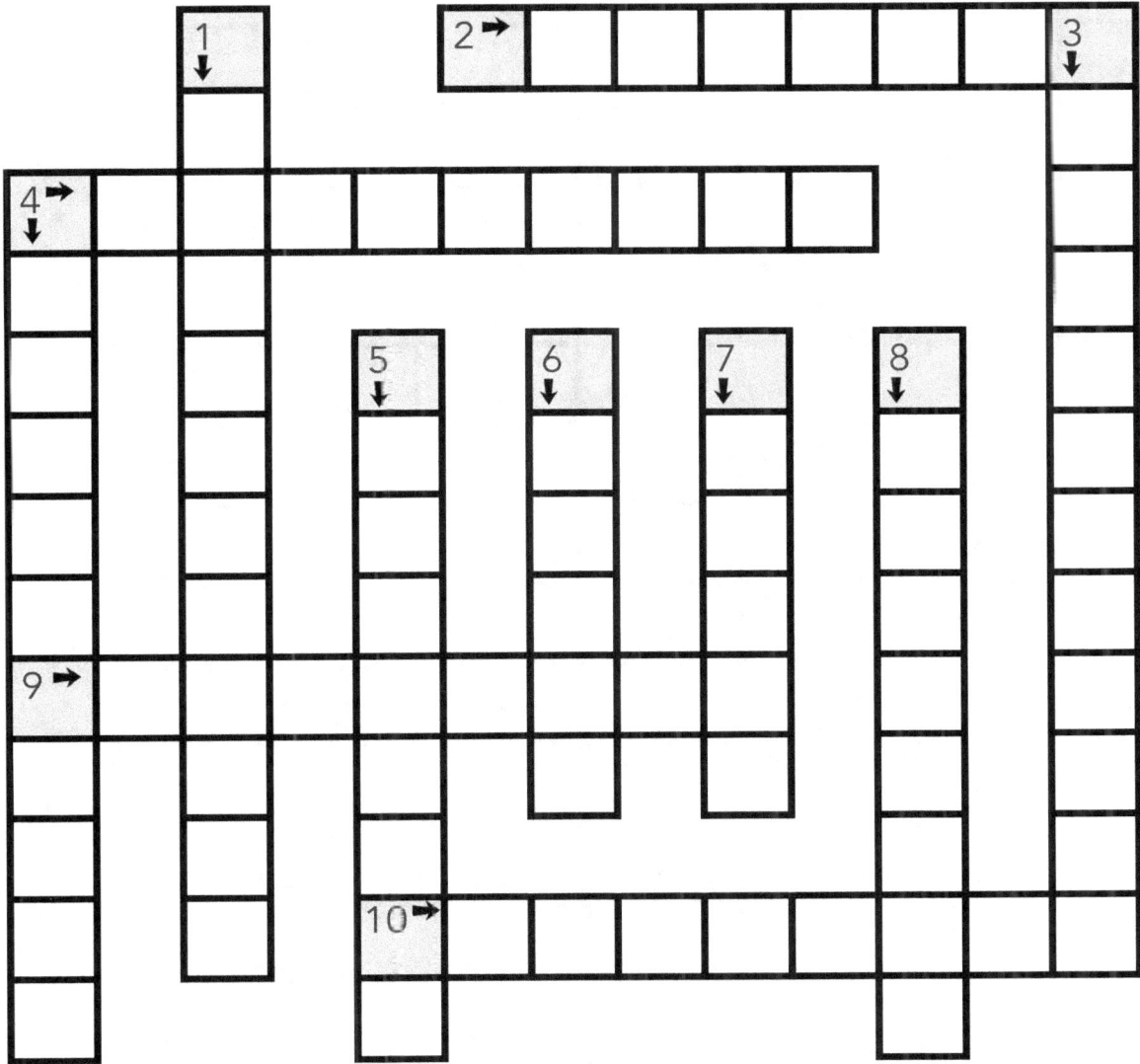

ACROSS
2. Malignant skin tumor from melanocytes.
4. Bacterial infection of deep skin layers.
9. Outermost layer of skin.
10. Chronic autoimmune skin condition.

DOWN
1. Inflammation of hair follicles.
3. Common inflammatory skin condition.
4. Treatment using extreme cold.
5. Light-based treatment for skin disorders.
6. Inflammatory skin condition causing itching.
7. Tissue sample extraction for examination.
8. Diagnostic method for skin allergies.

Solution on page 96

PUZZLE 05
ORTHOPEDICS

Medical Specialties

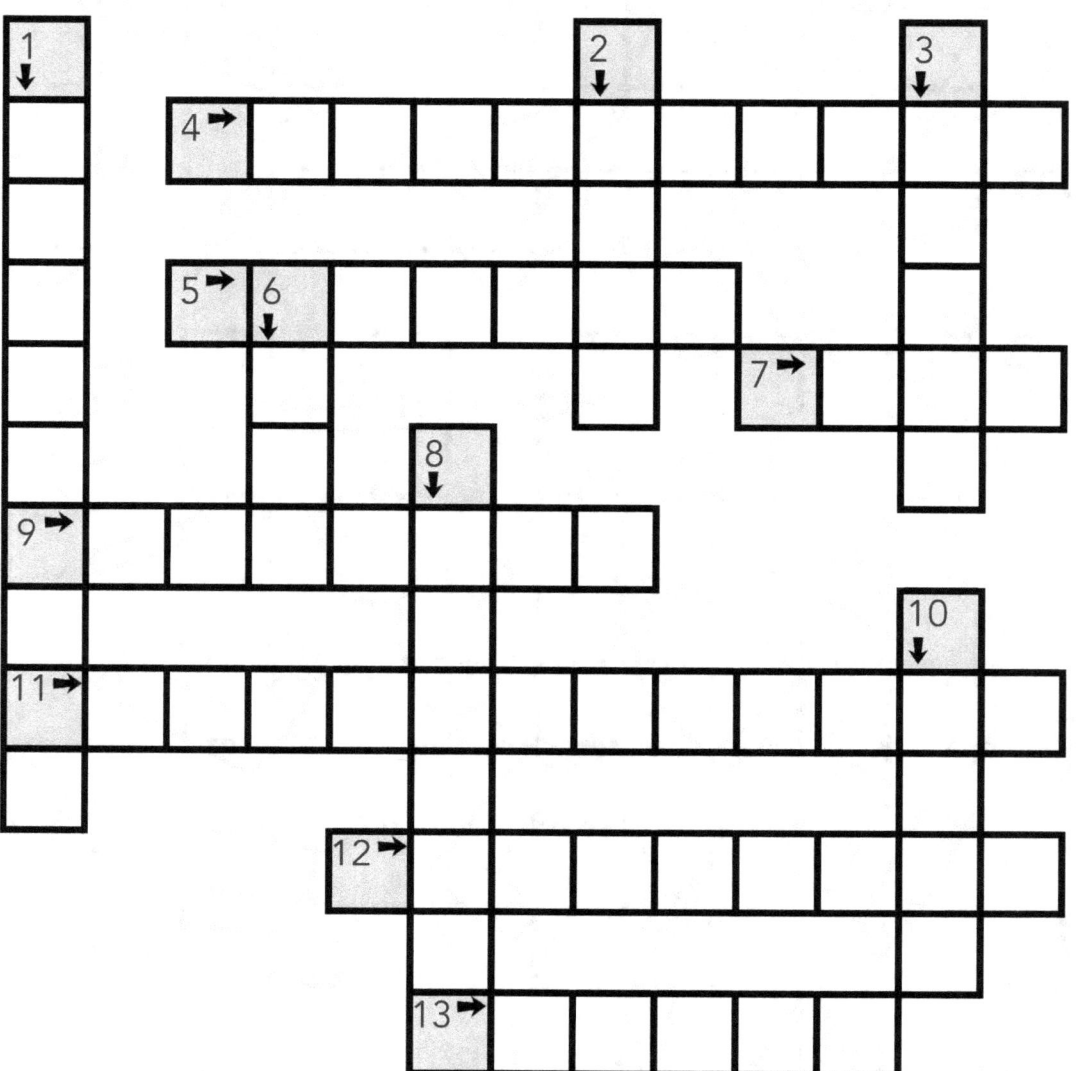

ACROSS
4. Skeletal strength measurement.
5. Upper arm long bone.
7. Skeletal imaging technique.
9. Connects bone to bone.
11. Joint lubricating substance.
12. Abnormal spinal curvature.
13. Temporary bone immobilization device.

DOWN
1. Bone-forming cell.
2. Longest bone in body.
3. Advanced cross-sectional imaging.
6. Forearm bone opposite radius.
8. Knee cartilage cushion.
10. Larger lower leg bone.

Solution on page 96

PUZZLE 06
GASTROENTEROLOGY

Medical Specialties

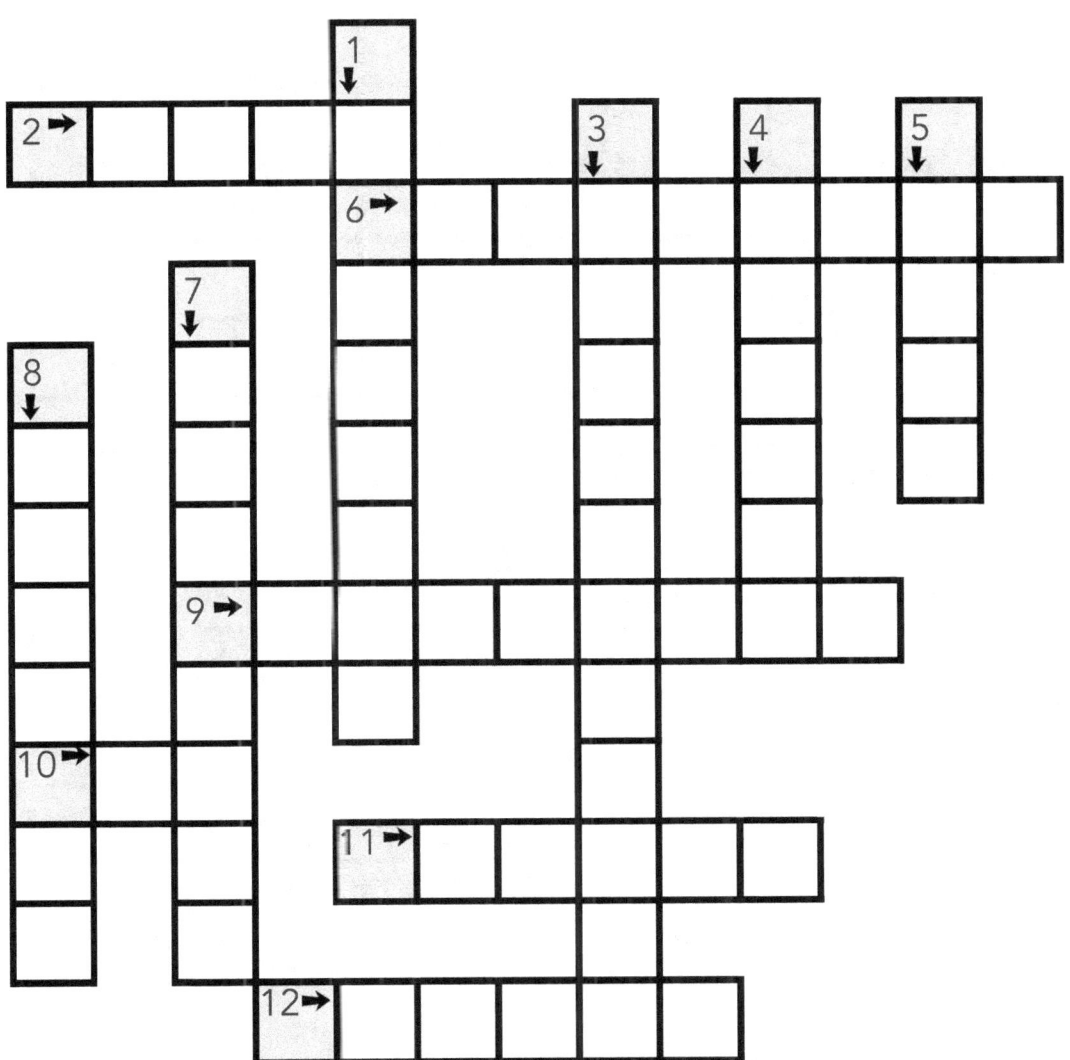

ACROSS

2. Large intestine segment absorbing water.
6. Upper abdominal discomfort or pain.
9. Liver inflammation, often viral.
10. Functional bowel disorder causing pain.
11. Final portion of digestive tract.
12. Tissue sample for diagnostic analysis.

DOWN

1. Internal organ examination via camera.
3. Appendix inflammation requiring surgery.
4. Stomach bacterium causing ulcers.
5. Vital organ performing metabolic functions.
7. Chronic liver scarring and dysfunction.
8. Yellowing of skin and eyes.

Solution on page 96

PUZZLE 07
PULMONOLOGY

Medical Specialties

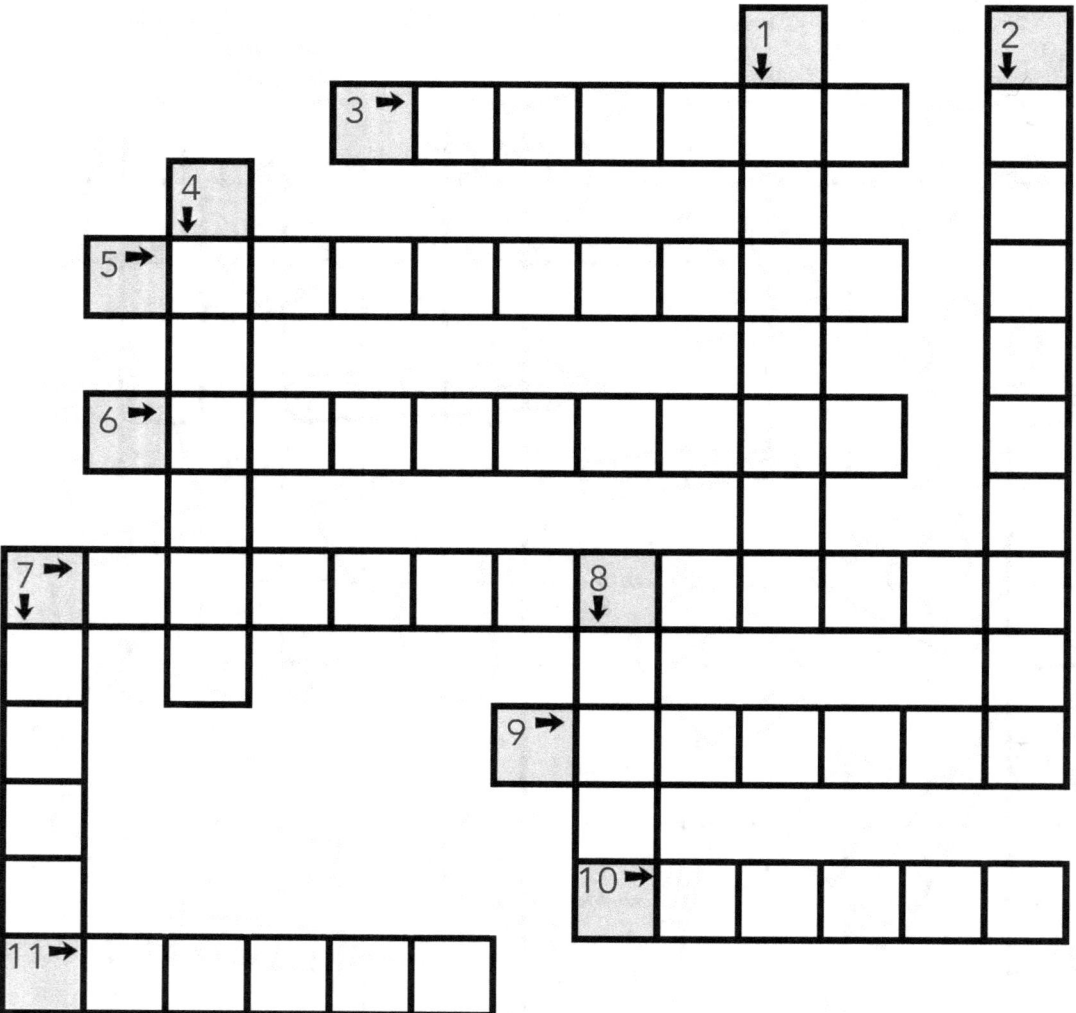

ACROSS

3. Airway branches in respiratory system.
5. Breathing pauses during sleep.
6. Coughing up blood.
7. Respiratory system specialist physician.
9. Medication delivery device for lungs.
10. Expelled mucus from respiratory tract.
11. Chronic airway inflammation condition.

DOWN

1. High-pitched breath sound.
2. Mechanical breathing assistance machine.
4. Tiny air sacs in lungs.
7. Membrane surrounding lungs.
8. Primary organs of respiration.

Solution on page 96

PUZZLE 08
ENDOCRINOLOGY

Medical Specialties

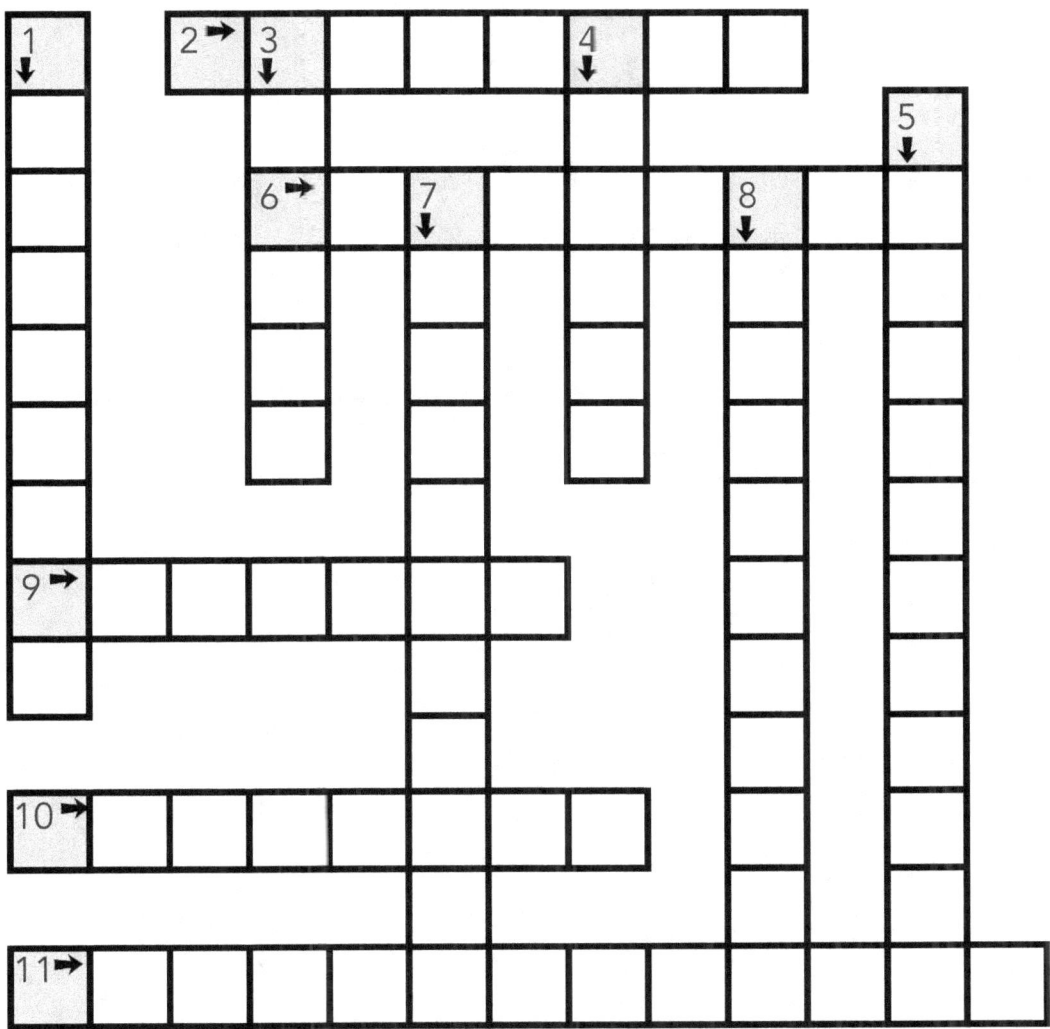

ACROSS

2. Hormone increasing blood glucose levels.
6. Master gland of endocrine system.
9. Blood sugar regulating pancreatic hormone.
10. Chronic condition affecting glucose metabolism.
11. Autoimmune thyroid disorder causing hyperthyroidism.

DOWN

1. Hormone stimulating milk production.
3. Hormone regulating energy balance, appetite.
4. Enlarged thyroid gland condition.
5. Brain region controlling endocrine function.
7. Inflammation of the thyroid gland.
8. Hormone regulating sodium and potassium.

Solution on page 97

PUZZLE 09
NEPHROLOGY

Medical Specialties

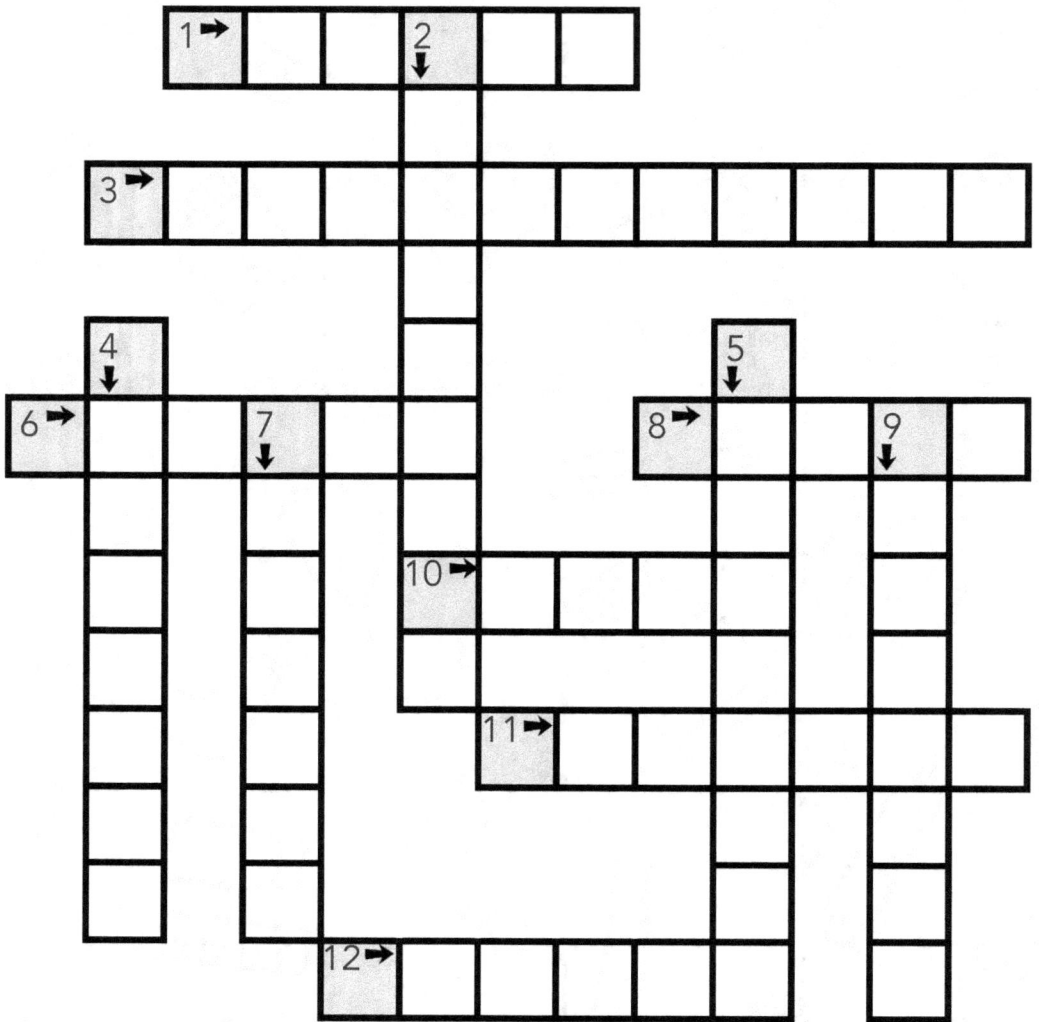

ACROSS

1. Tissue sample extraction for analysis.
3. Blood filtration treatment for kidneys.
6. Organ producing urine and hormones.
8. Pertaining to the kidneys.
10. Abnormal fluid accumulation in tissues.
11. Microscopic kidney structures for reabsorption.
12. Blood toxicity from kidney failure.

DOWN

2. Specialized cells in glomerular filtration.
4. Medication increasing urine production.
5. Presence of blood in urine.
7. Functional unit of the kidney.
9. Elevated nitrogen compounds in blood.

Solution on page 97

PUZZLE 10
RHEUMATOLOGY

Medical Specialties

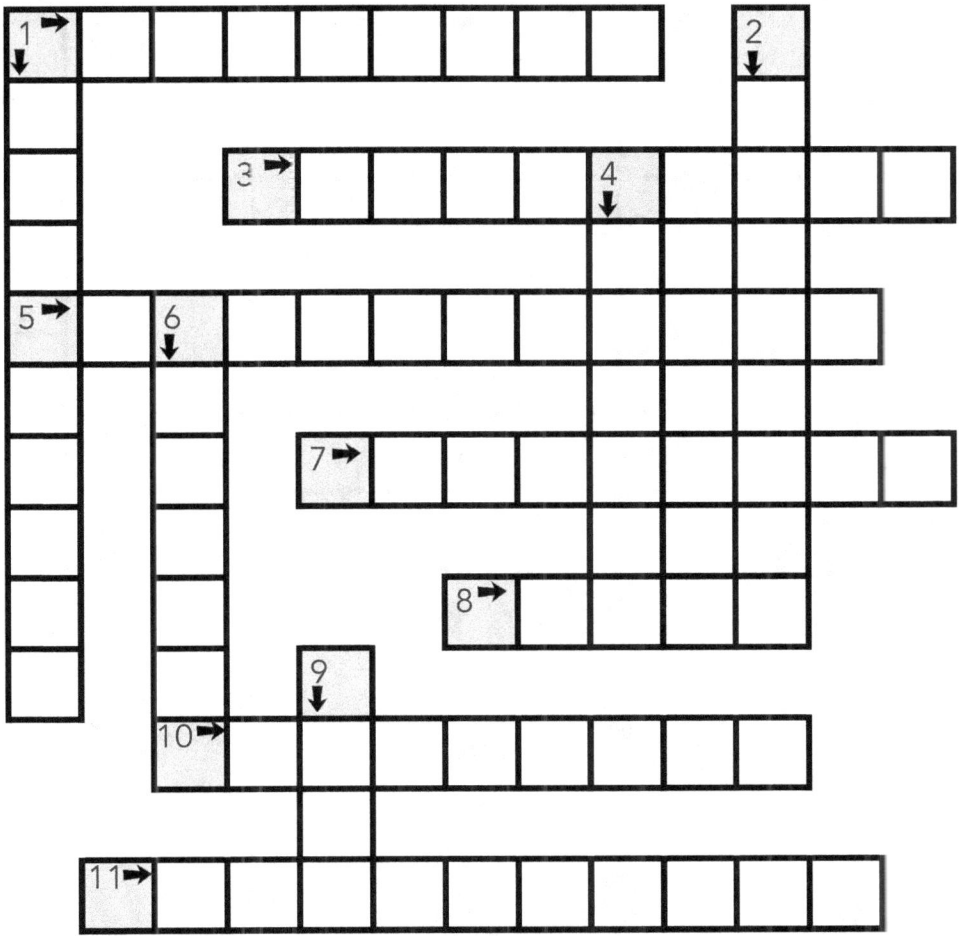

ACROSS

1. Joint disease causing pain and stiffness.
3. Chronic inflammatory disorder affecting multiple joints.
5. Tissue response to injury or infection.
7. Protein indicating presence of inflammation.
8. Autoimmune disease affecting multiple body systems.
10. Arthritis associated with skin condition.
11. Red blood cell carrying oxygen.

DOWN

1. Immune system attacking body's own tissues.
2. Genetically engineered drugs targeting immune system.
4. Antibody test for rheumatoid arthritis.
6. Sudden worsening of symptoms.
9. Painful arthritis caused by uric acid.

Solution on page 97

PUZZLE 11
OPHTHALMOLOGY

Medical Specialties

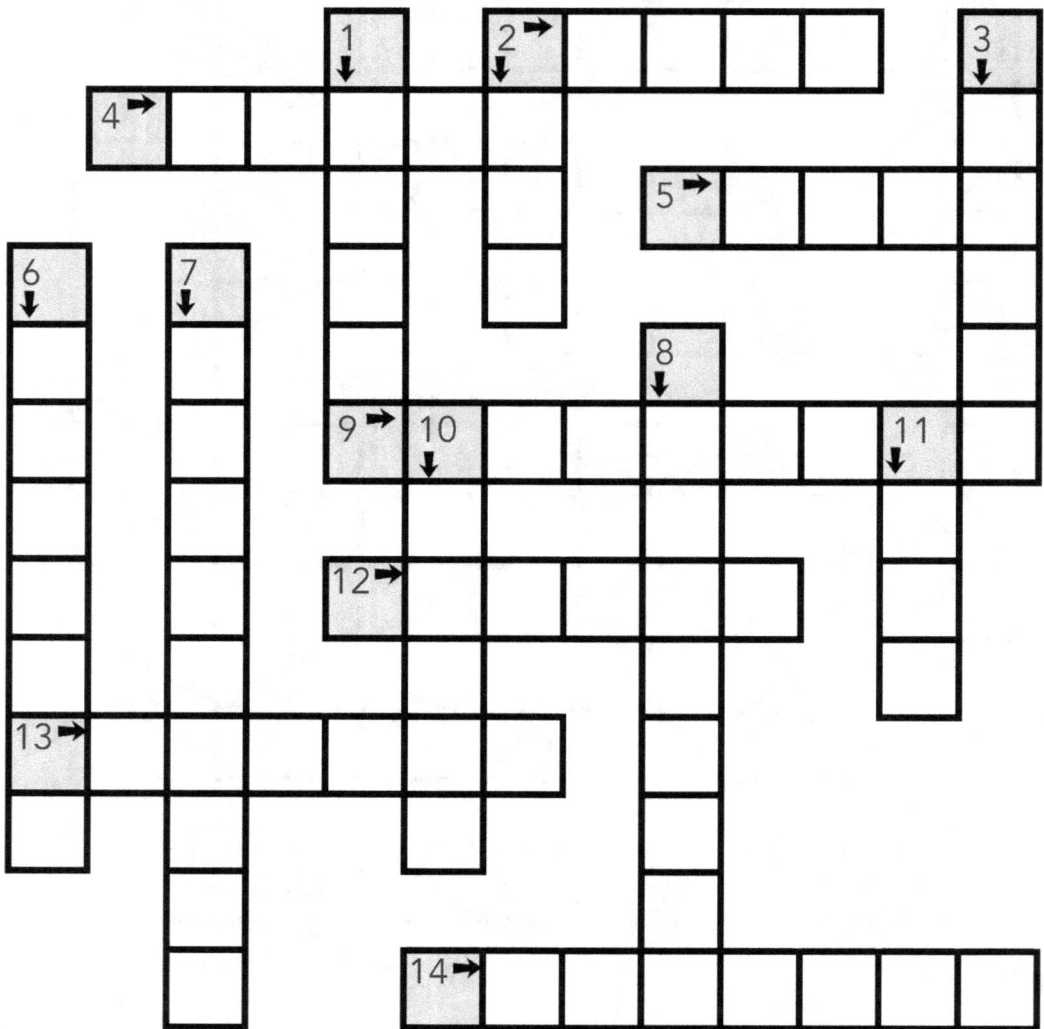

ACROSS

2. Refractive surgery using excimer laser.
4. Insufficient tear production condition.
5. Light-regulating ocular aperture.
9. Reduced vision from childhood.
12. Transparent anterior eye surface.
13. Inflammation of eye's middle layer.
14. Clouding of eye's natural lens.

DOWN

1. Light-sensitive tissue lining eye.
2. Focusing structure behind iris.
3. Protective white outer eye layer.
6. Gel-like substance filling eyeball.
7. Visual information pathway to brain.
8. Difficulty focusing on near objects.
10. Nearsightedness requiring corrective lenses.
11. Colored eye part controlling light.

Solution on page 97

PUZZLE 12
OTOLARYNGOLOGY (ENT)

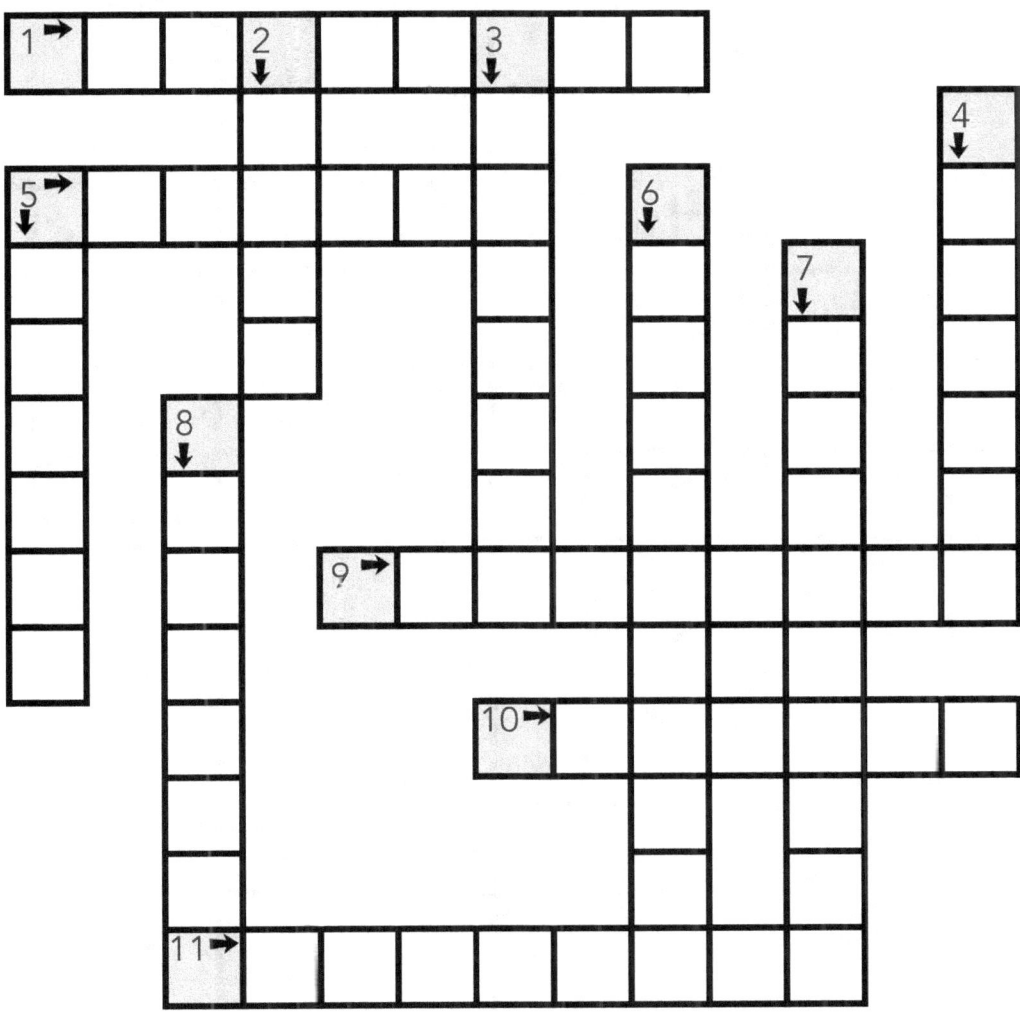

ACROSS

1. Inflammation of paranasal sinus cavities.
5. Waxy substance in ear canal.
9. Difficulty producing normal vocal sounds.
10. Sensation of spinning or dizziness.
11. Bleeding from the nasal passages.

DOWN

2. Fleshy extension hanging from soft palate.
3. Perception of ringing in ears.
4. Loss of sense of smell.
5. Spiral-shaped inner ear structure.
6. Upper part of the throat.
7. Inflammation of the voice box.
8. Instrument for examining ear canal.

PUZZLE 13
HEMATOLOGY

Medical Specialties

ACROSS
1. Oxygen-carrying blood cells.
5. Liquid component of blood.
9. Blood cells aiding clotting.
10. Low red blood cell condition.
11. Process stopping blood loss.

DOWN
2. Inherited hemoglobin disorder.
3. Genetic blood clotting deficiency.
4. Cancer of blood-forming tissues.
6. Anticoagulant medication.
7. Undifferentiated progenitor cells.
8. Red blood cell destruction.

Solution on page 97

PUZZLE 14
PEDIATRICS

Medical Specialties

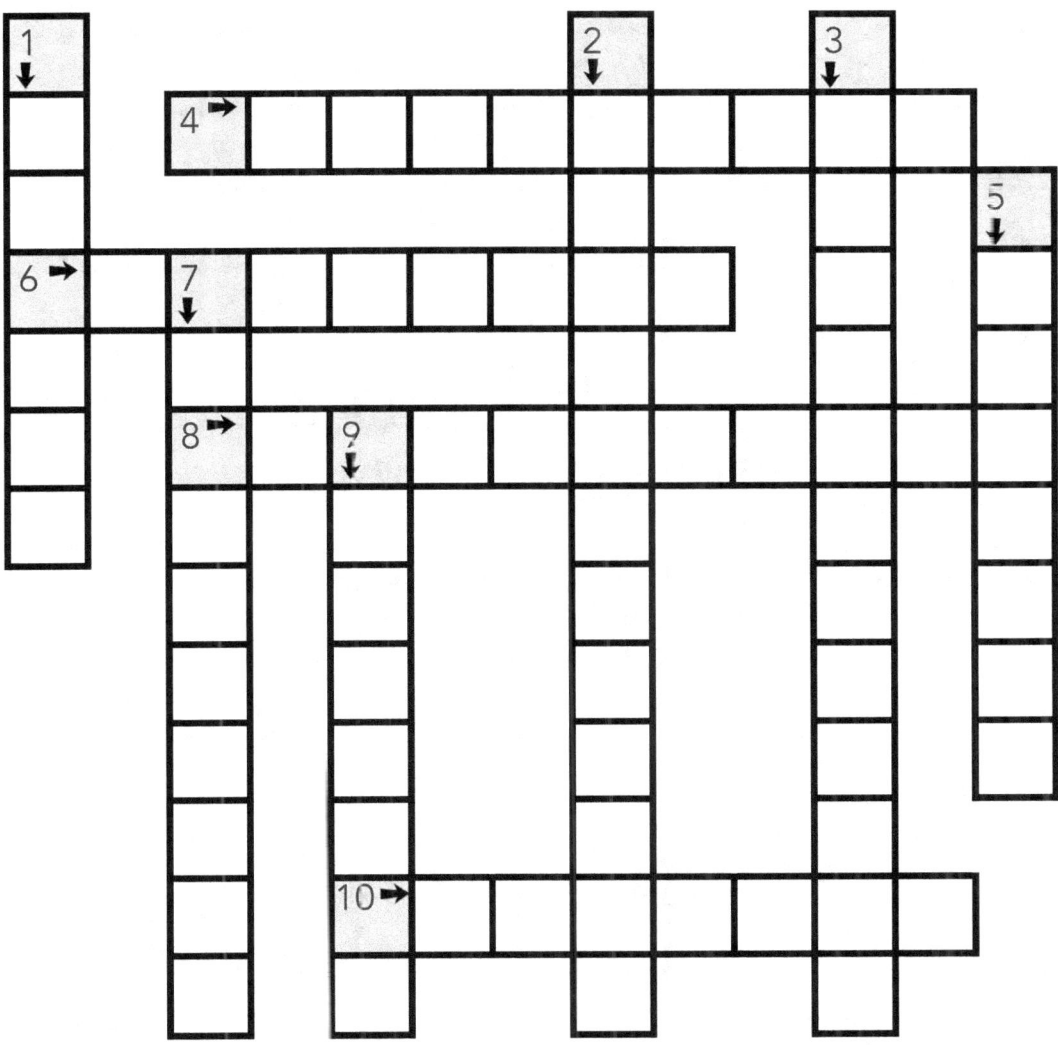

ACROSS

4. Irritated skin in infant's diaper area.
6. Wrapping technique for newborn comfort.
8. Pediatric tool tracking physical development.
10. Infant soothing device for suckling.

DOWN

1. Highly contagious viral exanthem disease.
2. Lower respiratory tract inflammation in infants.
3. Portable medication delivery device for bronchodilation.
5. Eruption process of primary dentition.
7. Newborn health assessment at birth.
9. Instrument for examining ear canal.

Solution on page 97

PUZZLE 15
GERIATRICS

Medical Specialties

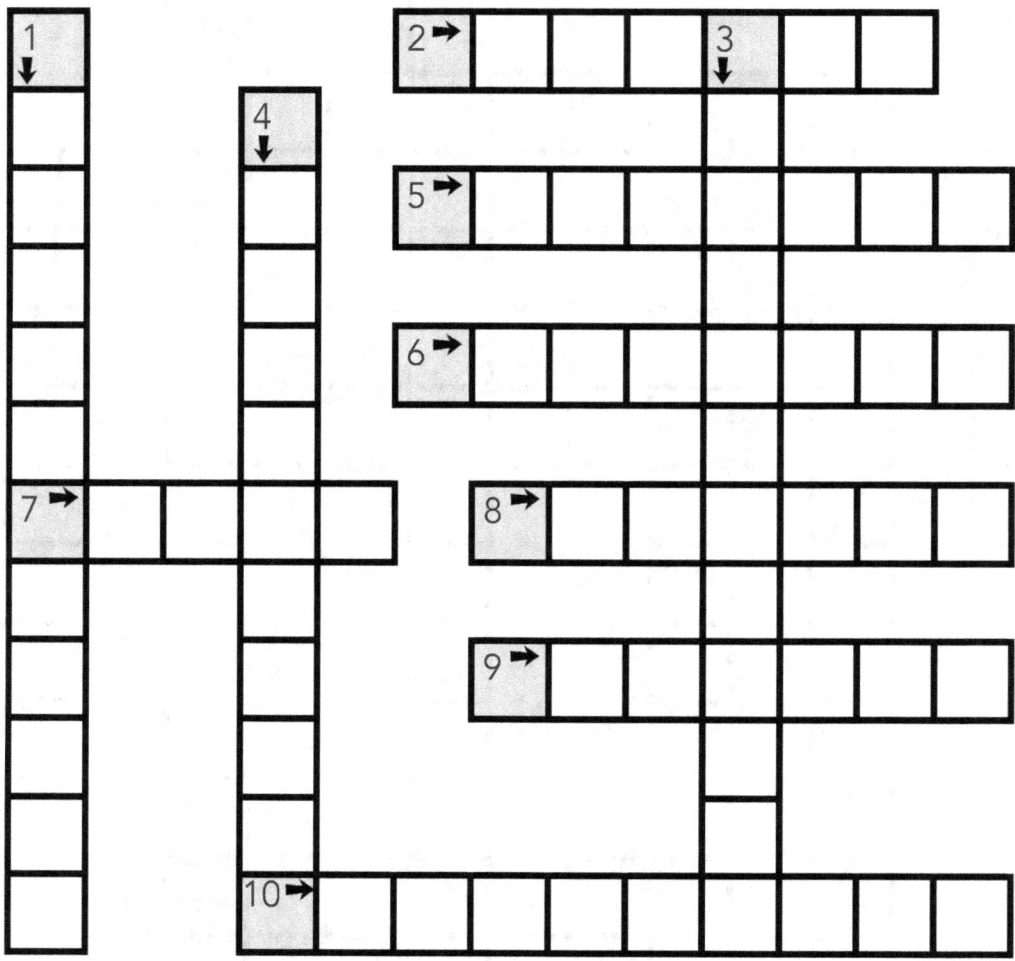

ACROSS

2. End-of-life care facility.
5. Federal health insurance for seniors.
6. Progressive cognitive decline disorder
7. Biological process of growing older.
8. Decreased physiological reserve and resilience.
9. Advanced age population group.
10. Age-related loss of muscle mass.

DOWN

1. Concurrent use of multiple medications.
3. Involuntary loss of bladder control.
4. Decreased auditory perception ability.

Solution on page 97

PUZZLE 16
Obstetrics and Gynecology (OB-GYN)

Medical Specialties

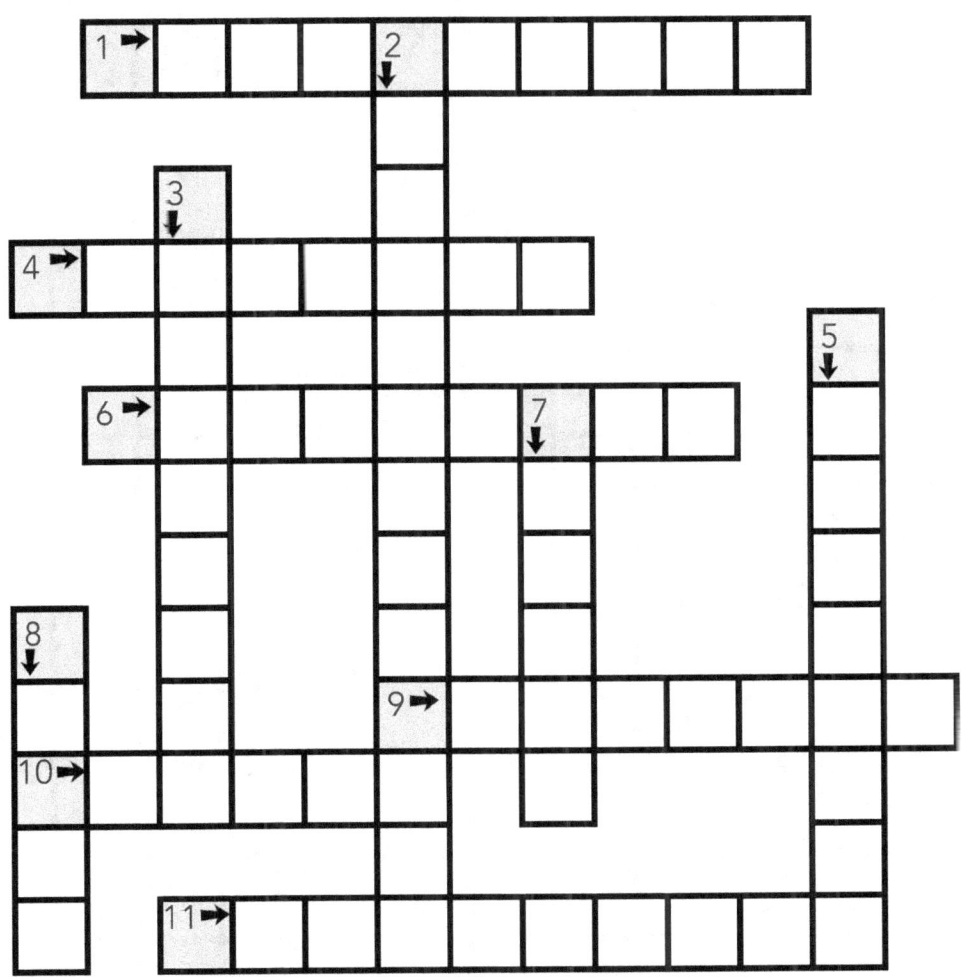

ACROSS

1. Imaging technique using high-frequency sound waves.
4. Surgical delivery through abdominal incision.
6. Essential B vitamin for fetal development.
9. Spinal anesthesia for pain management.
10. Hollow organ for fetal development.
11. Surgical incision to aid childbirth.

DOWN

2. Prenatal test of amniotic fluid.
3. Cessation of menstrual cycles.
5. Gestation period of fetal development.
7. Lower part of the uterus.
8. Non-medical birth support professional.

Solution on page 98

PUZZLE 17
PSYCHIATRY

Medical Specialties

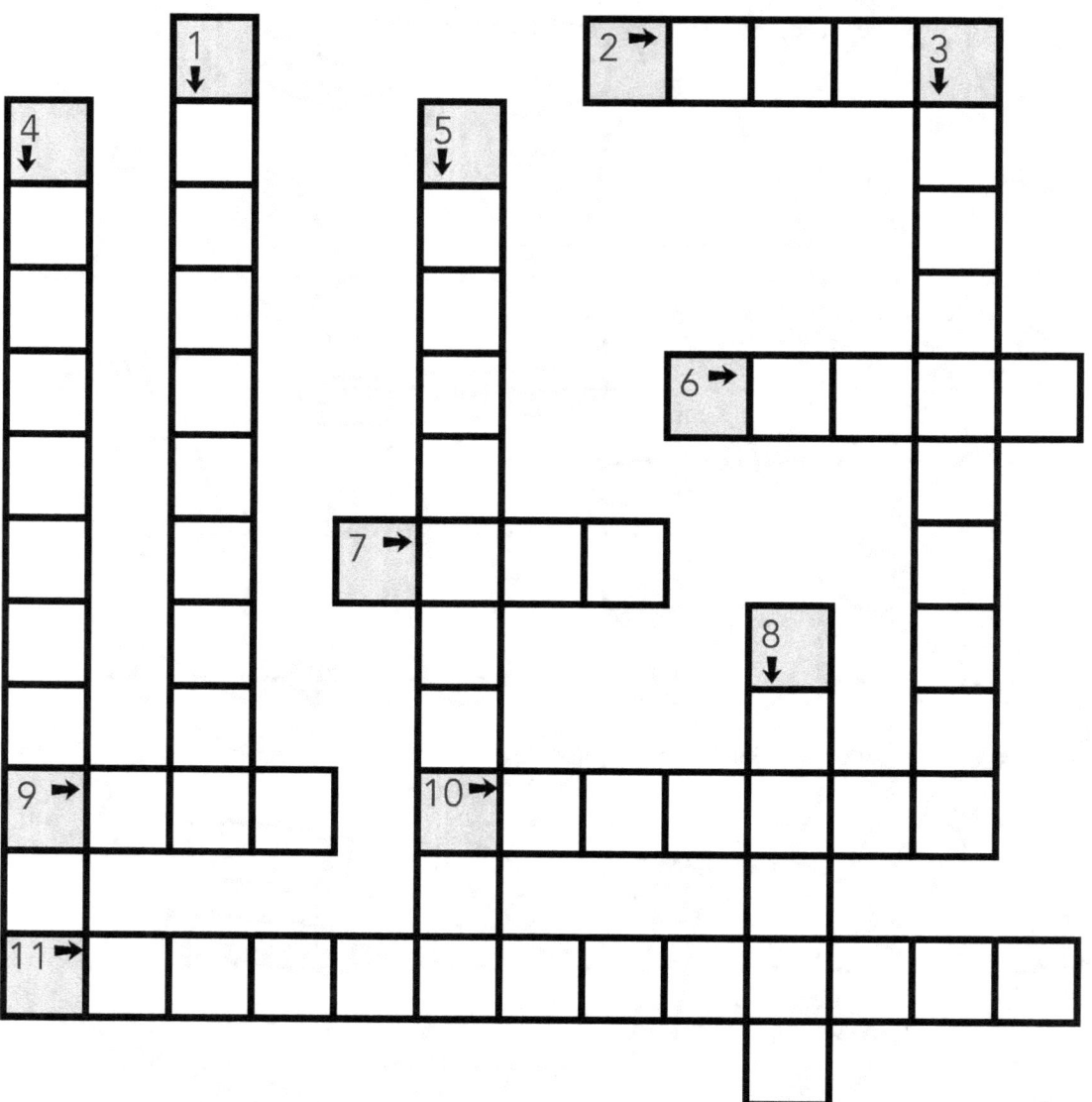

ACROSS

2. Psychoanalysis pioneer.
6. Individual psychology founder.
7. Collective unconscious theorist.
9. Cognitive therapy developer.
10. Psychosocial development stages theorist.
11. Severe mental illness medication.

DOWN

1. Anxiety-reducing drug.
3. Mood disorder with persistent sadness.
4. Fear of open or crowded spaces.
5. Present-moment awareness practice.
8. Hierarchy of needs psychologist.

Solution on page 98

PUZZLE 18
RADIOLOGY

Medical Specialties

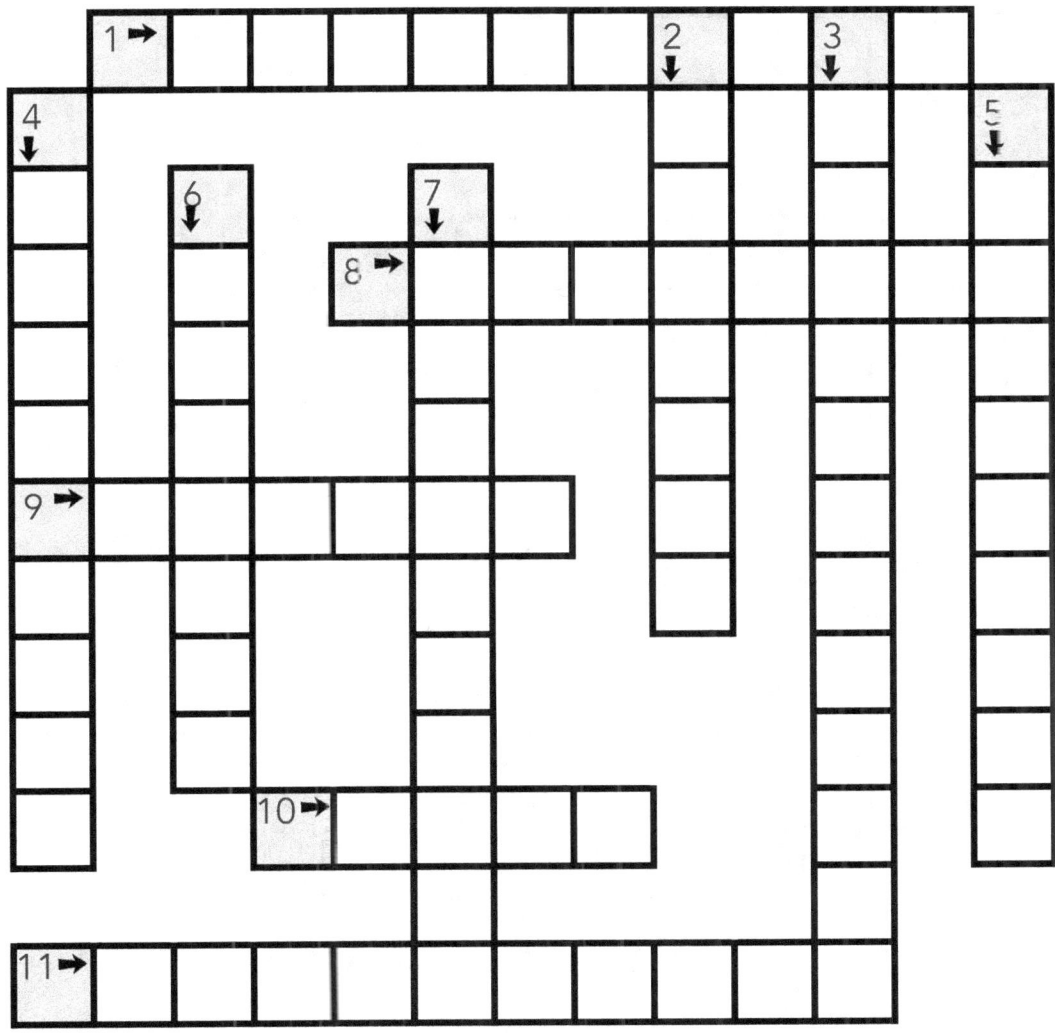

ACROSS

1. Measure of skeletal mineral content.
8. Breast tissue imaging examination.
9. Metabolic activity imaging technique.
10. Nuclear medicine 3D imaging method.
11. Emitting ionizing radiation spontaneously.

DOWN

2. Diagnostic ultrasound imaging procedure.
3. Iodine absorption measurement test.
4. Impenetrable by X-rays or radiation.
5. Sectional imaging of body tissues.
6. Unit of radiation exposure measurement.
7. Nuclear medicine imaging device.

Solution on page 98

PUZZLE 19
ANESTHESIOLOGY

Medical Specialties

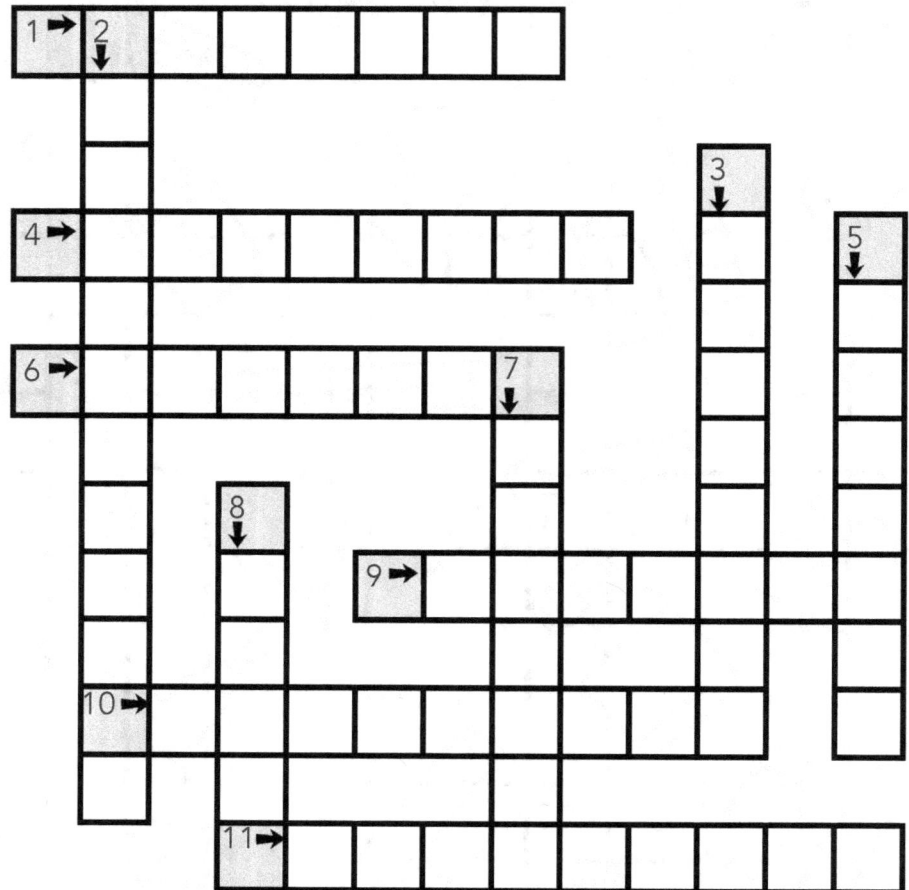

ACROSS

1. Intravenous anesthetic for rapid induction.
4. Benzodiazepine used for preoperative anxiolysis.
6. Dissociative anesthetic with analgesic properties.
9. Pharmacologically induced state of calm.
10. Volatile halogenated ether anesthetic agent.
11. Rapid-onset inhalational anesthetic gas.

DOWN

2. Ultra-short-acting synthetic opioid analgesic.
3. Local anesthetic and antiarrhythmic drug.
5. Potent synthetic opioid pain medication.
7. Neuraxial analgesia technique for labor.
8. Narcotic class of pain-relieving drugs.

Solution on page 98

24

PUZZLE 20
UROLOGY

Medical Specialties

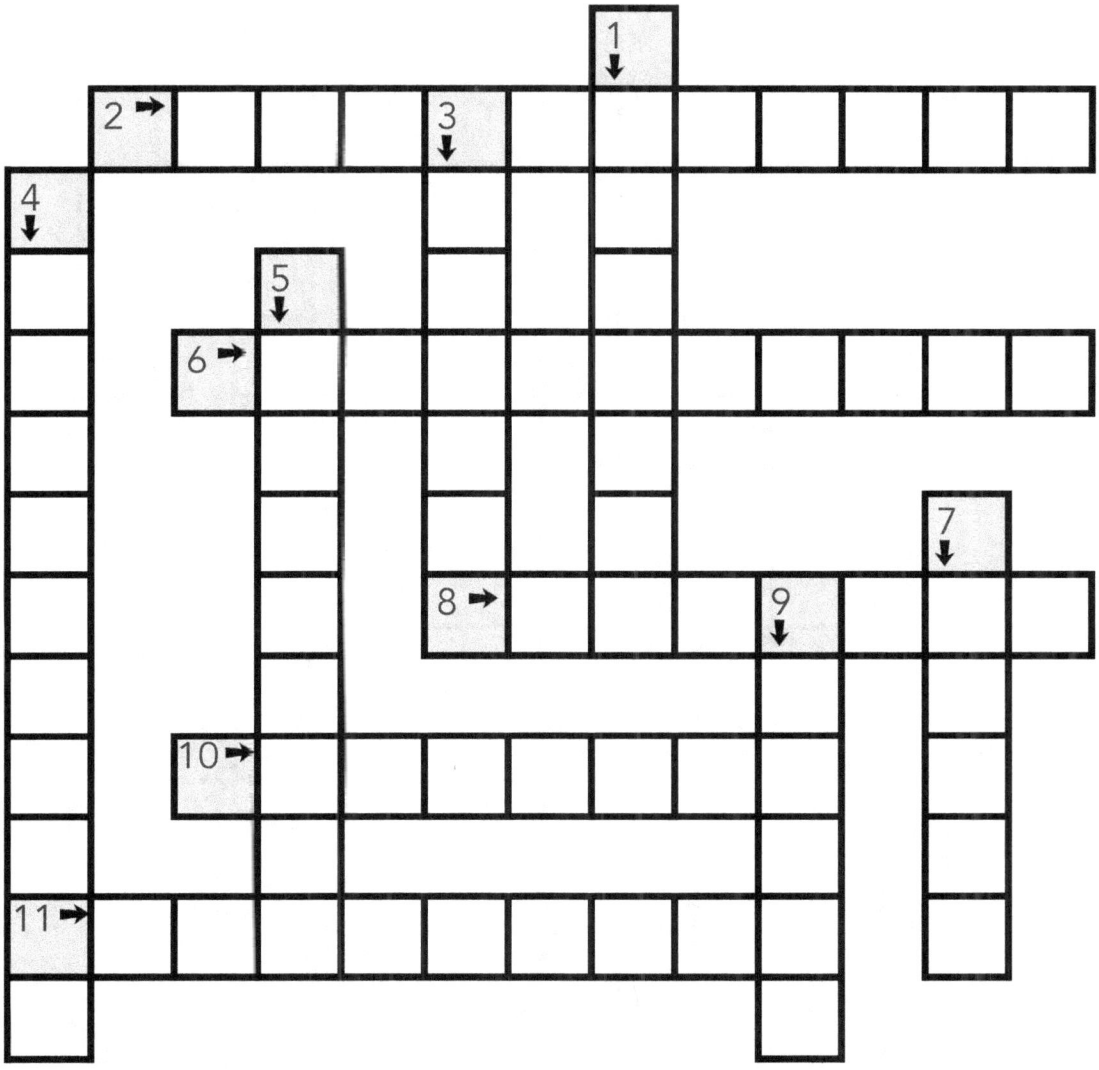

ACROSS
2. Involuntary loss of bladder control.
6. Surgical removal of a kidney.
8. Excessive urination during night.
10. Male gland surrounding urethra.
11. Waste product measured in urine.

DOWN
1. Medication promoting urine production.
3. Functional unit of the kidney.
4. Study of bladder and urethra function.
5. Blood present in urine.
7. Organ filtering blood and producing urine.
9. Tube carrying urine to bladder.

Solution on page 98

PUZZLE 21
INFECTIOUS DISEASES

Medical Specialties

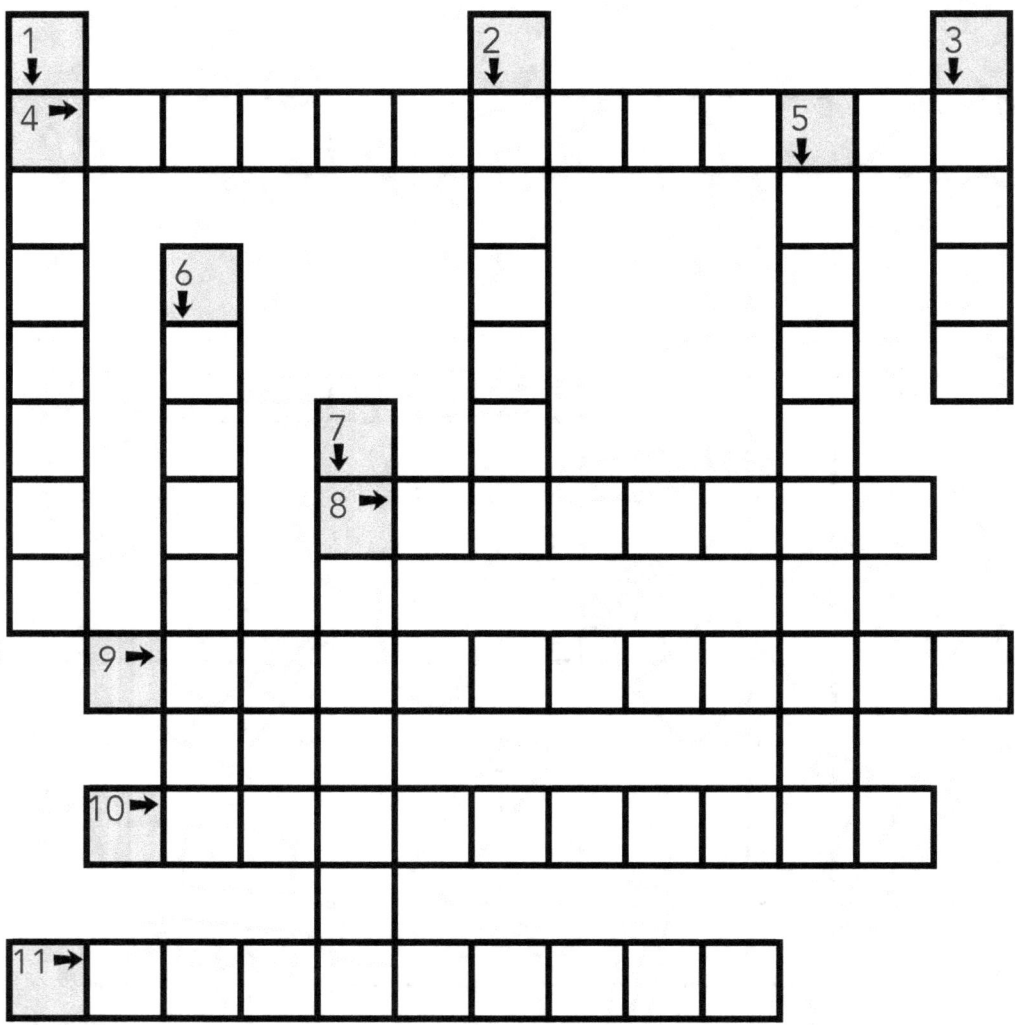

ACROSS
4. Inhibits or destroys microorganisms.
8. Sudden occurrence of disease cases.
9. Disease spread between individuals.
10. Pathogen carried by organism.
11. Originating in healthcare setting.

DOWN
1. Disease spreading across continents.
2. Nucleic acid amplification technique.
3. Antibody detection immunoassay method.
5. Pathogen development before symptoms.
6. Spreading through air particles.
7. Transmitted from animals to humans.

Solution on page 98

PUZZLE 22
IMMUNOLOGY

Medical Specialties

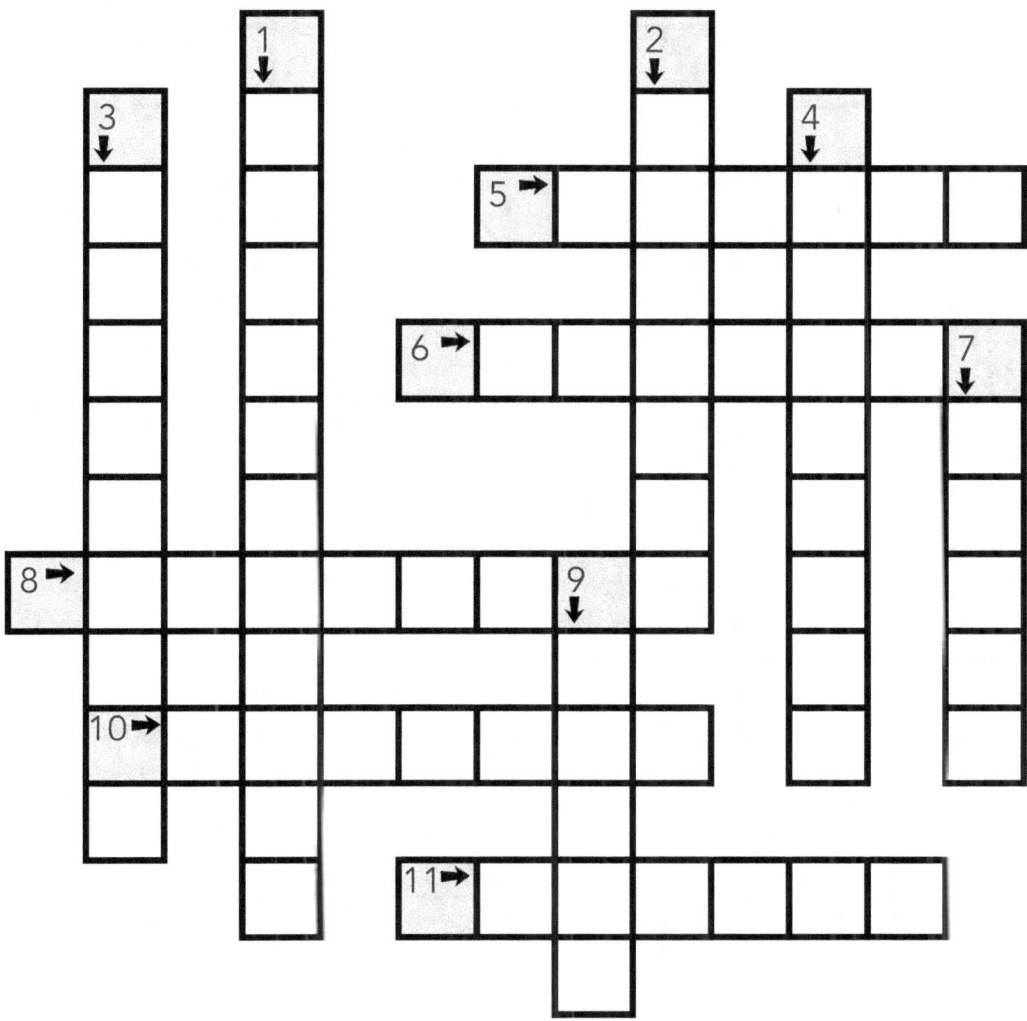

ACROSS

5. Lymphocytes with innate cytotoxic function.
6. Molecules triggering immune responses.
8. Substances enhancing vaccine efficacy.
10. Specific antibody binding sites.
11. Hypersensitivity to environmental substances.

DOWN

1. Population-wide disease resistance.
2. Preparations stimulating immune protection.
3. Proteins neutralizing foreign substances.
4. Substances provoking allergic reactions.
7. Lymphoid organ filtering blood.
9. Lymphocytes mediating cellular immunity.

Solution on page 98

PUZZLE 23
PATHOLOGY

Medical Specialties

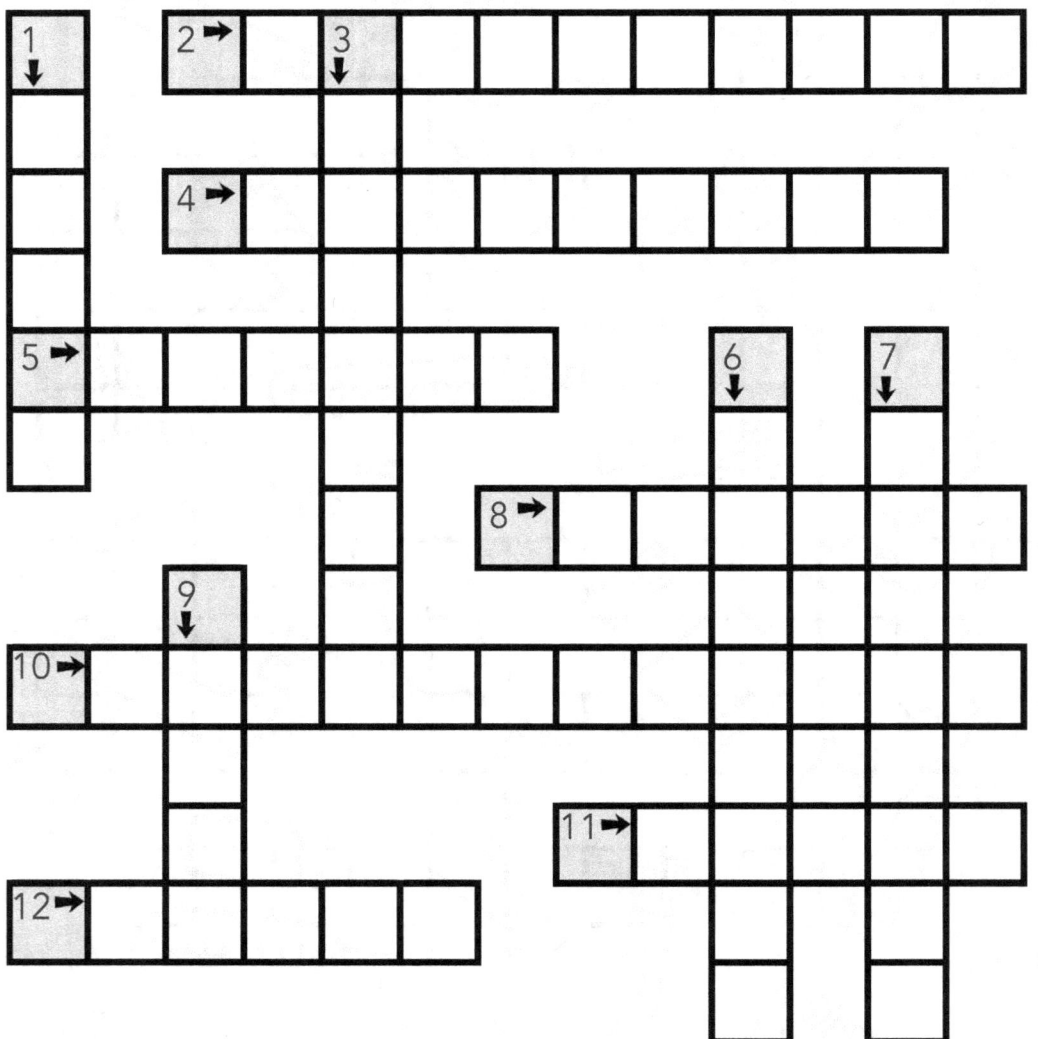

ACROSS

2. Nuclear stain in tissue preparation.
4. Magnification tool for cellular examination.
5. Malignant tumor of connective tissue.
8. Post-mortem examination of body.
10. Rapid intraoperative tissue analysis.
11. Abnormal change in tissue structure.
12. Non-cancerous growth or tumor type.

DOWN

1. Tissue sample for diagnostic analysis.
3. Instrument for thin tissue sectioning.
6. Programmed cell death process.
7. Study of tissue microanatomy.
9. Cytoplasmic stain in tissue preparation.

Solution on page 98

PUZZLE 24
PLASTIC SURGERY

Medical Specialties

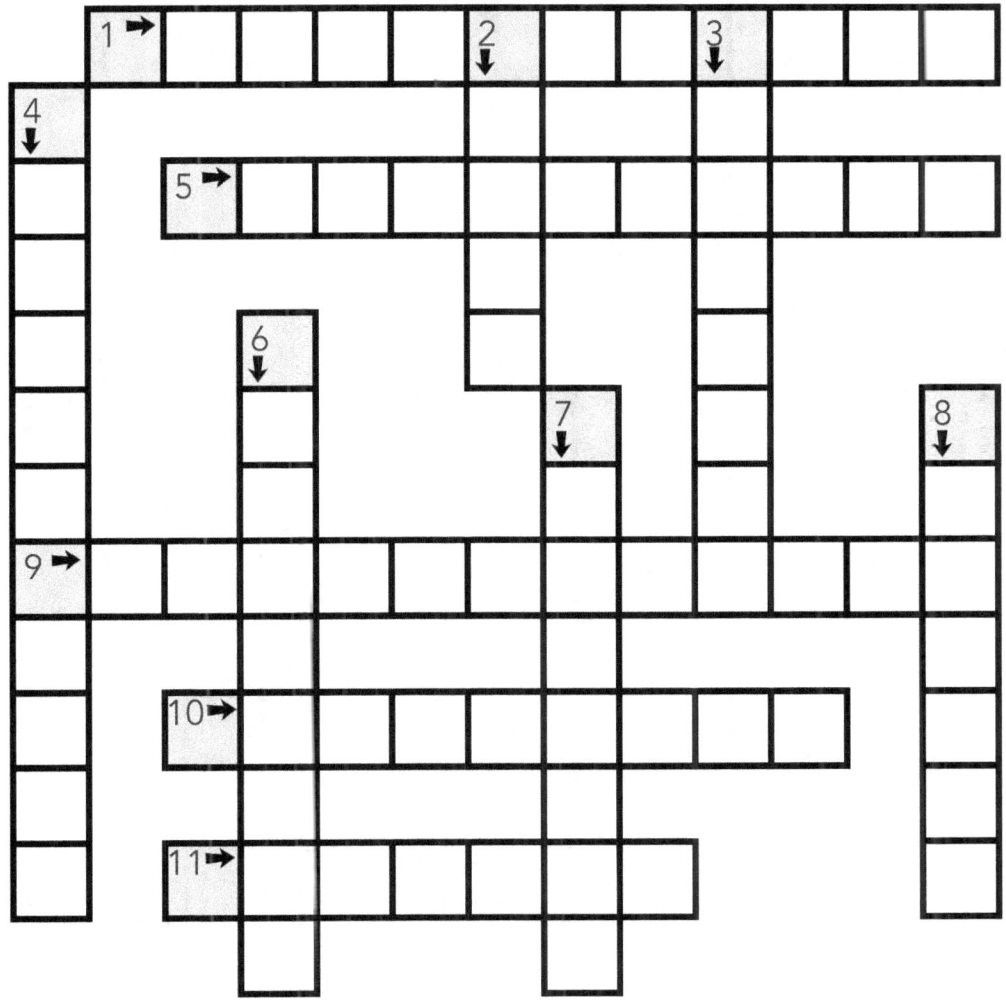

ACROSS
1. Skin resurfacing technique using abrasive tool.
5. Congenital oral cavity malformation.
9. Skin exfoliation using acidic solutions.
10. Surgical correction of prominent ears.
11. Precise surgical cutting instrument.

DOWN
2. Neurotoxin for wrinkle reduction injections.
3. Implant material for augmentation procedures.
4. Fat removal through suction technique.
6. Abdominal contouring surgical procedure.
7. Protein for dermal filler injections.
8. Rhinoplasty procedure for nasal reshaping.

Solution on page 99

PUZZLE 25
EMERGENCY MEDICINE

Medical Specialties

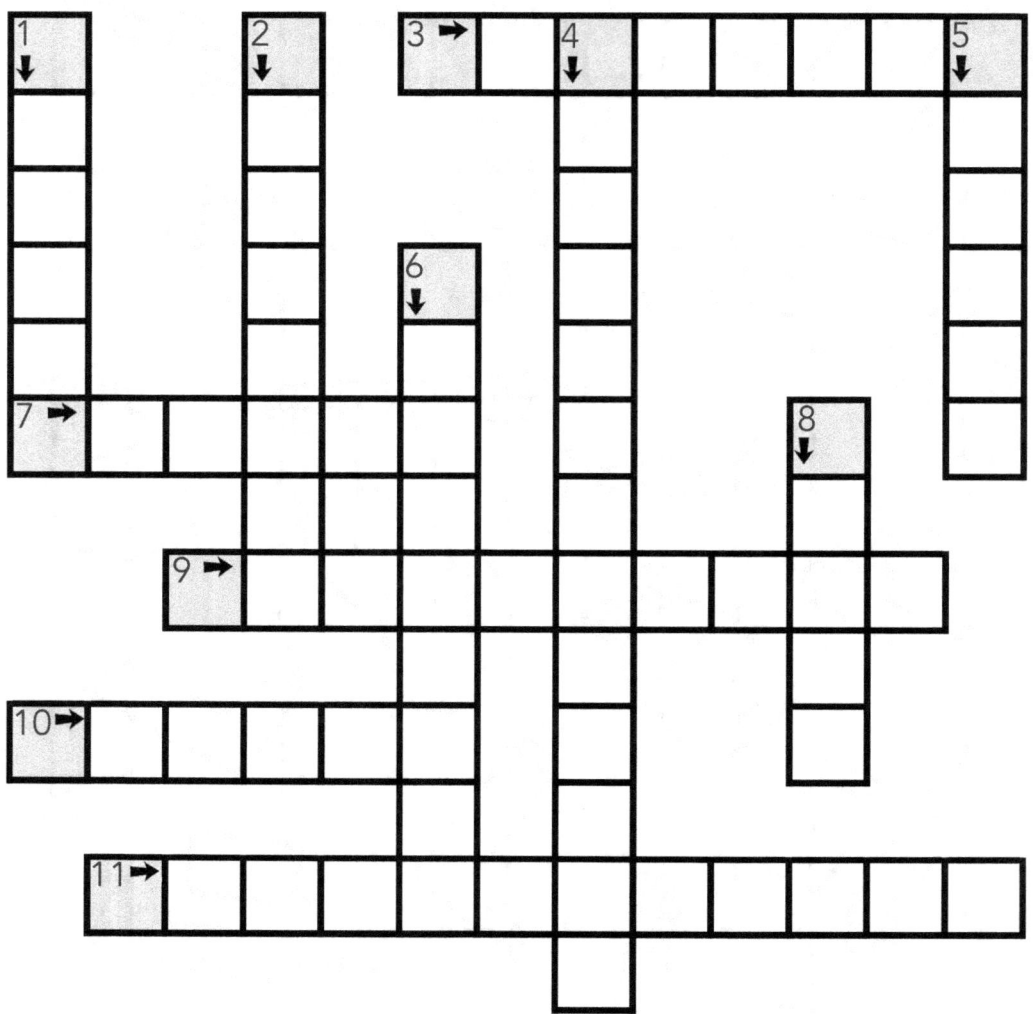

ACROSS

3. Emergency resuscitation team activation protocol.
7. Cerebrovascular event causing neurological deficits.
9. Mechanical breathing assistance device.
10. Physical injury requiring immediate intervention.
11. Instrument for visualizing vocal cords.

DOWN

1. Systemic inflammatory response to infection.
2. Excessive intake of drugs/substances.
4. Device delivering electrical shock to heart.
5. Epinephrine auto-injector for anaphylaxis.
6. Symptom suggesting cardiac distress.
8. Inadequate tissue perfusion and oxygenation.

Solution on page 99

PUZZLE 26
NOBEL PRIZE IN MEDICINE

Medical Generalities and Miscellaneous

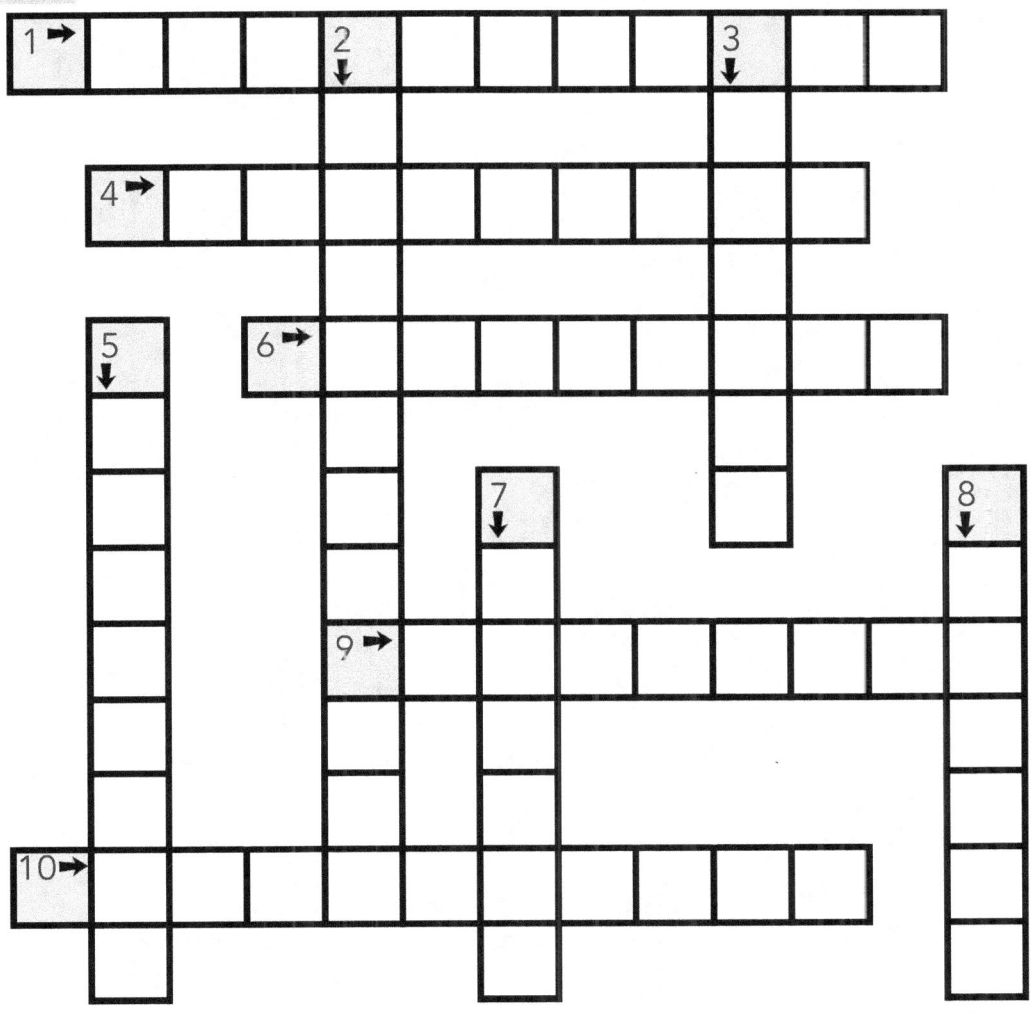

ACROSS

1. Biological process of chromosome replication and cytoplasmic separation.
4. Viral infection affecting the liver, discovered in 1989.
6. Undifferentiated cells capable of developing into specialized cell types.
9. Protective structures at chromosome ends, linked to cellular aging.
10. Technique for modifying DNA sequences in living organisms.

DOWN

2. Molecular configuration of genetic material, elucidated by Watson and Crick.
3. Pancreatic hormone regulating glucose metabolism.
5. Genes with potential to cause cancer when mutated or over-expressed.
7. Parasitic disease transmitted by Anopheles mosquitoes.
8. French microbiologist who developed the process of pasteurization.

Solution on page 99

PUZZLE 27
FAMOUS MEDICAL DISCOVERIES

Medical Generalities and Miscellaneous

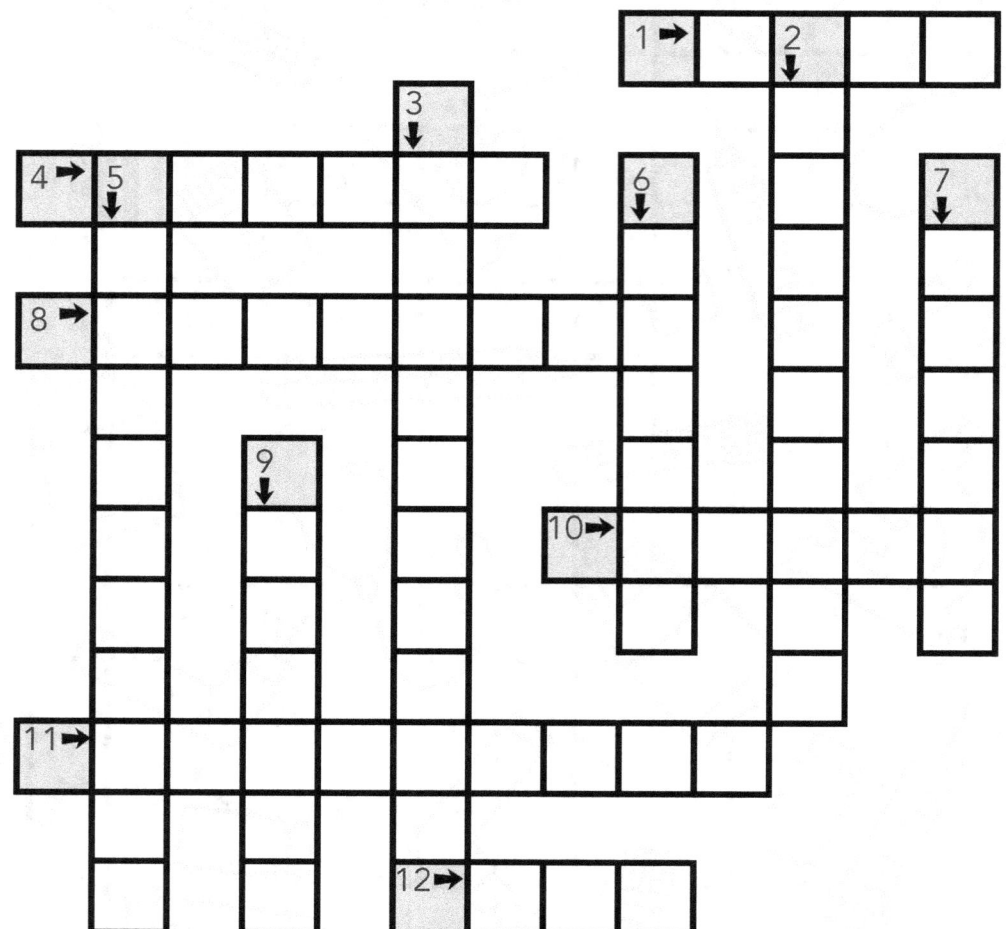

ACROSS

1. Röntgen's electromagnetic radiation discovery.
4. Germ theory and vaccination pioneer.
8. Multipotent cell research breakthrough.
10. Surgical antisepsis innovator.
11. van Leeuwenhoek's magnification invention.
12. Polio vaccine developer.

DOWN

2. Lister's wound infection prevention method.
3. Koch's bacillus identification.
5. Fleming's penicillin discovery.
6. Banting and Best's diabetes treatment.
7. First human heart transplant surgeon.
9. Hoffman's pain relief medication synthesis.

Solution on page 99

PUZZLE 28
ANCIENT MEDICINE

Medical Generalities and Miscellaneous

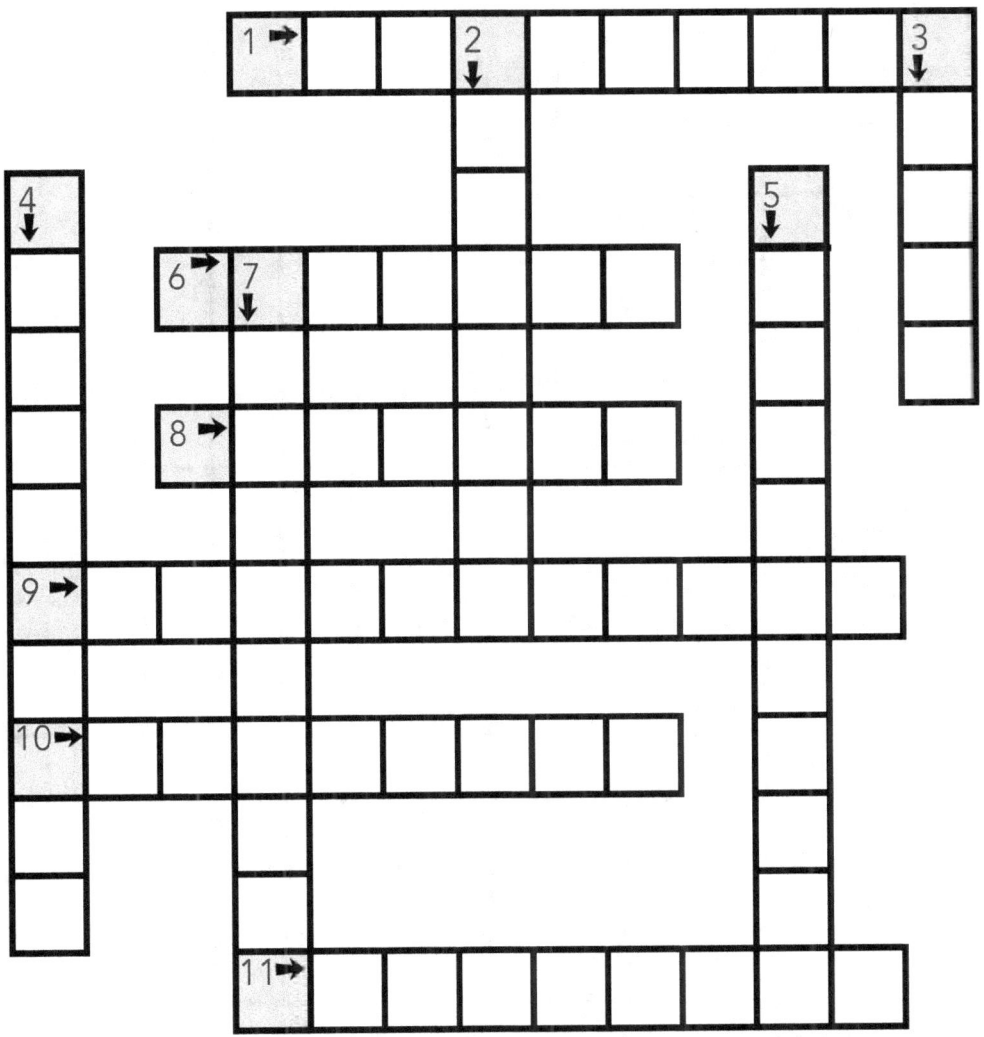

ACROSS

1. Ancient Chinese complementary forces concept.
6. Divine intervention healing practice.
8. Protective talismans in folk medicine.
9. Ancient Egyptian medical text.
10. Greek god of healing.
11. Energy pathways in traditional acupuncture.

DOWN

2. Traditional Indian holistic medicine system.
3. Influential Roman physician and anatomist.
4. Medieval pharmacy or pharmacist.
5. Herb-burning therapeutic technique.
7. Four bodily fluids health theory.

Solution on page 99

PUZZLE 29
MEDICAL PIONEERS

Medical Generalities and Miscellaneous

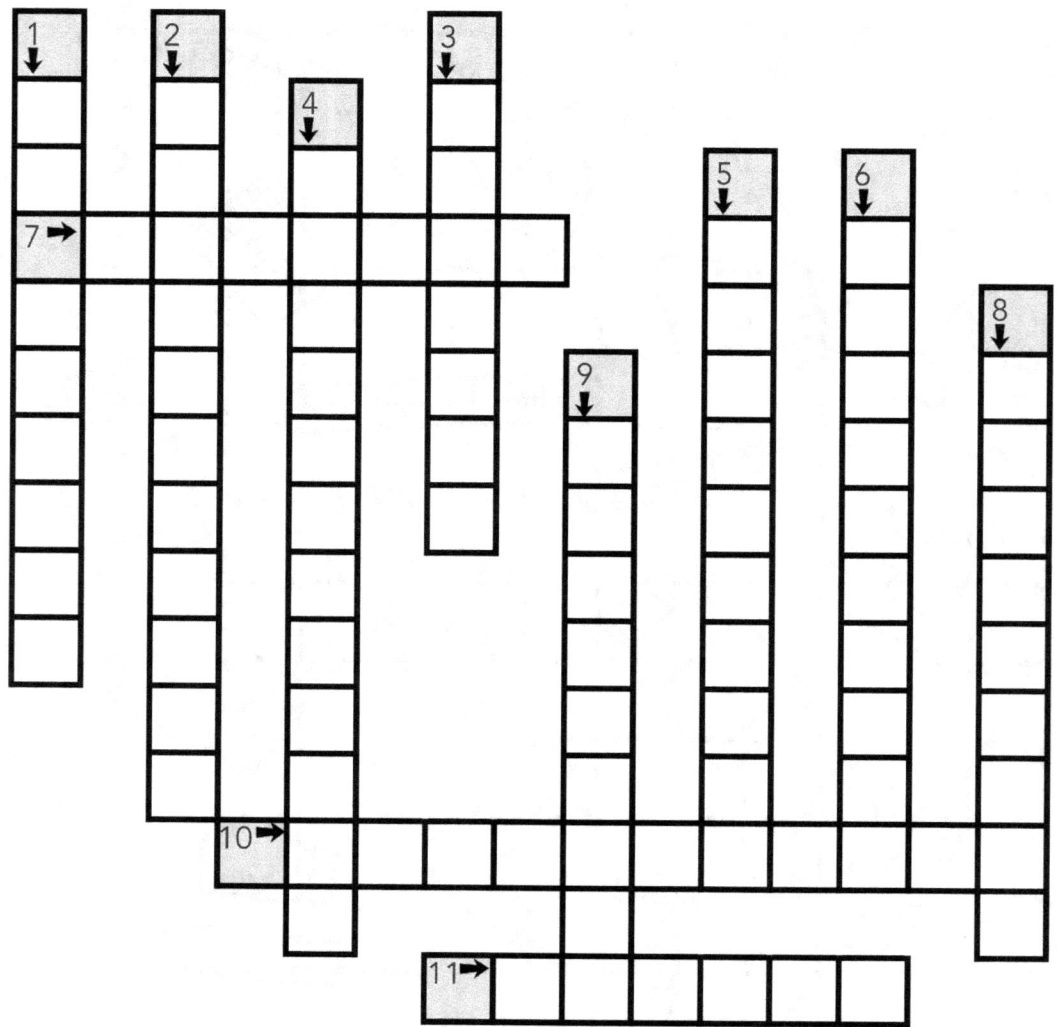

ACROSS
7. Jenner's vaccination target.
10. Germ theory pioneer.
11. Banting and Best's diabetes treatment.

DOWN
1. Morton's pain-relieving innovation.
2. Cowpox inoculation developer.
3. Controversial psychosurgical procedure.
4. Ether anesthesia demonstrator.
5. Ancient Greek "Father of Medicine".
6. Laennec's chest examination tool.
8. Pasteur's microorganism disease concept.
9. Landsteiner's transfusion compatibility discovery.

Solution on page 99

PUZZLE 30
MEN'S HEALTH

Medical Generalities and Miscellaneous

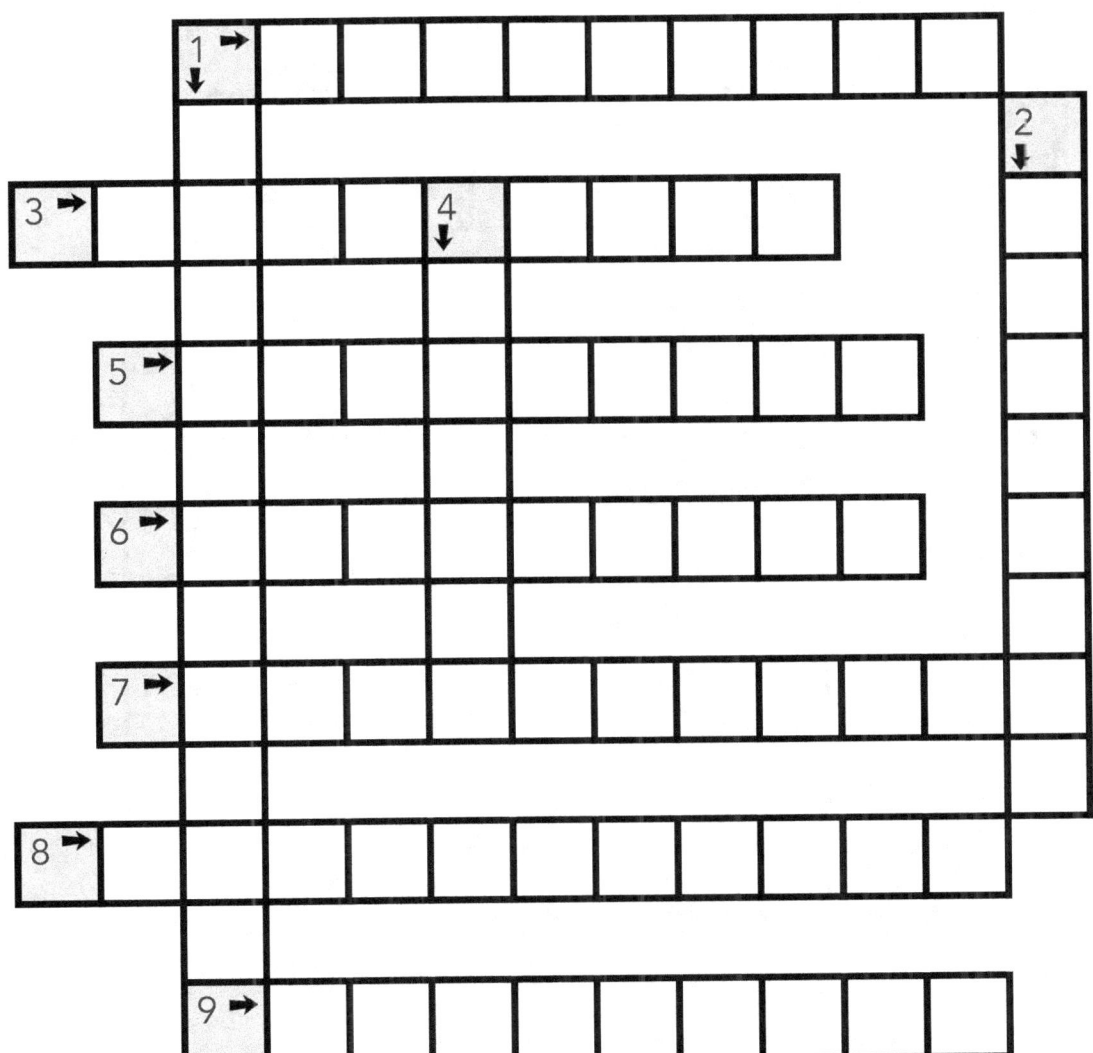

ACROSS

1. Lean tissue targeted in resistance training.
3. Male hormonal decline with aging.
5. Visible rectus abdominis musculature.
6. Mood disorder affecting mental health.
7. Digital rectal screening procedure.
8. Primary male sex hormone.
9. Breathing disorder during slumber.

DOWN

1. Emotional transition in middle age.
2. Male sterilization surgical procedure.
4. Prostate-specific antigen screening method.

Solution on page 99

PUZZLE 31
MEDICAL DEVICES

Medical Generalities and Miscellaneous

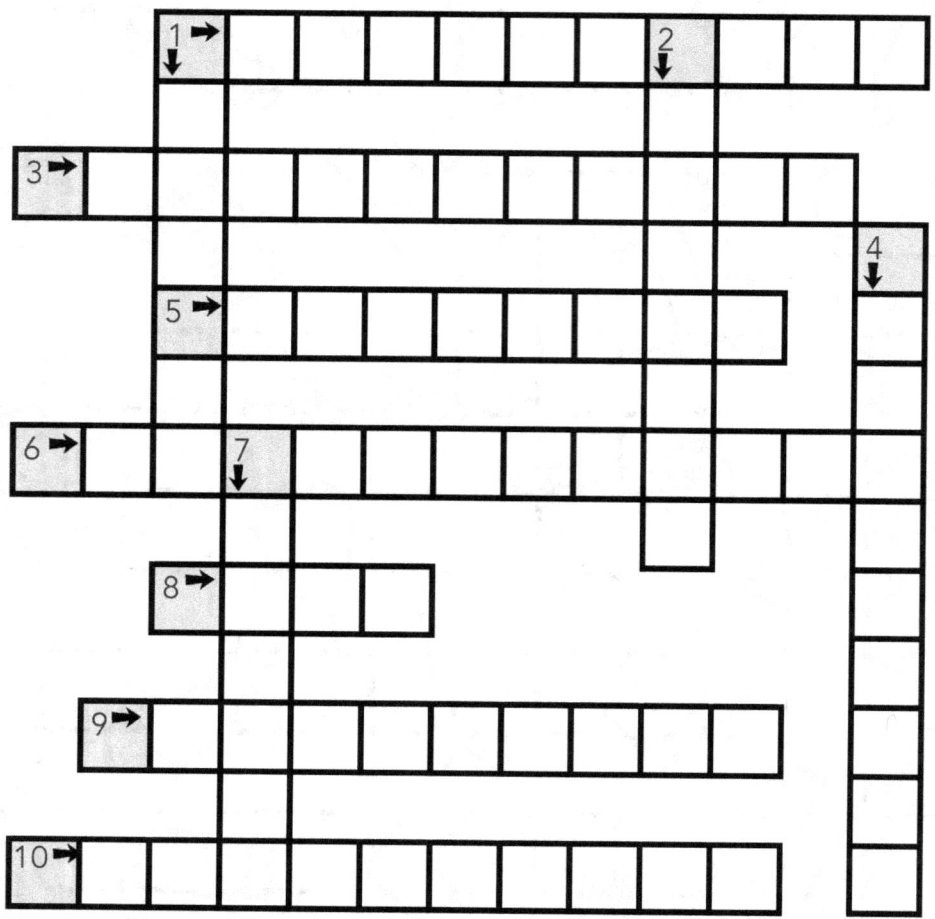

ACROSS

1. Auscultation device for listening to body sounds.
3. Cardiac electrical activity tracking apparatus.
5. Implantable cardiac rhythm regulation device.
6. Peripheral oxygen saturation measurement instrument.
8. Electromagnetic radiation imaging system.
9. Mechanical respiratory support machine.
10. Mobility assistance devices for non-ambulatory patients.

DOWN

1. Surgical incision instrument with sharp blade.
2. Tubular medical device for fluid drainage.
4. Auditory amplification device for hearing-impaired.
7. Fluid injection or aspiration instrument.

Solution on page 99

PUZZLE 32
SURGICAL TECHNIQUES

Medical Generalities and Miscellaneous

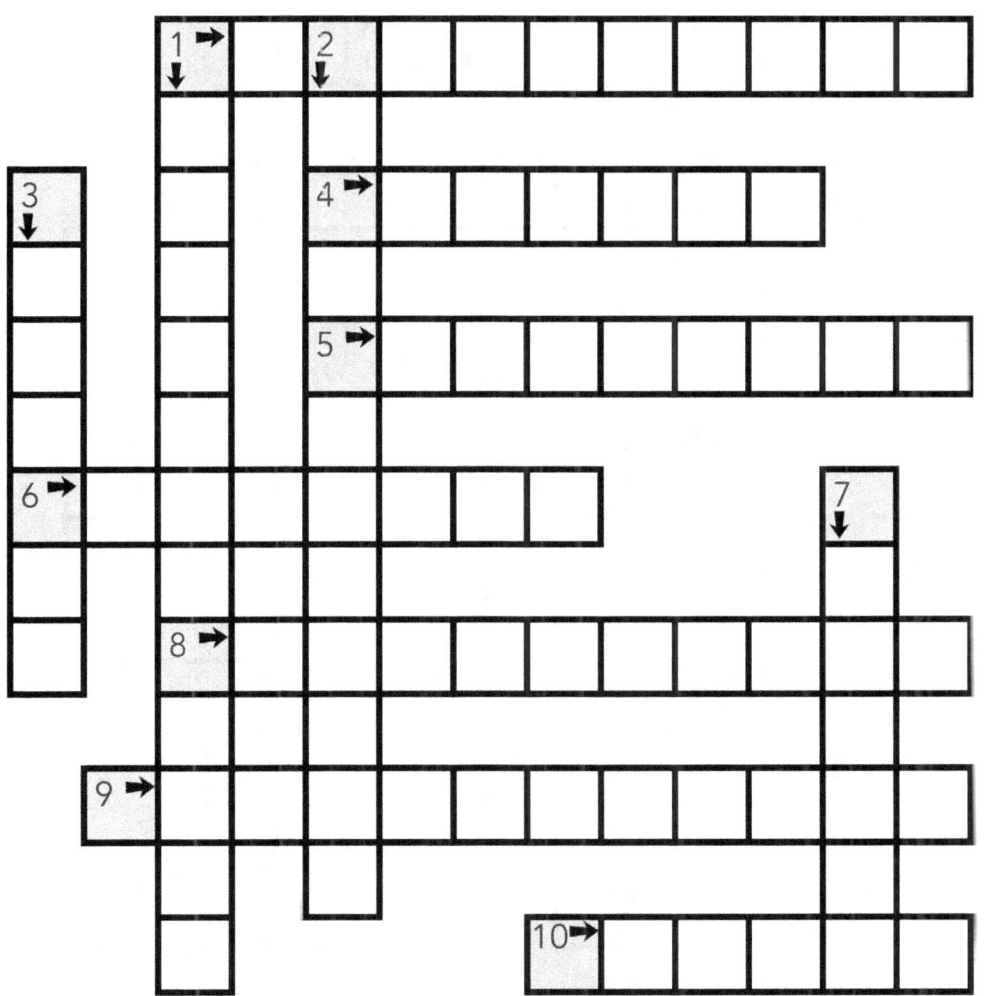

ACROSS

1. Endoscopic examination of large intestine.
4. Sharp surgical cutting instrument.
5. Tool to hold tissue open.
6. Spinal anesthetic injection technique.
8. Blood vessel widening procedure.
9. Precision operations using microscope.
10. Tissue sample extraction for analysis.

DOWN

1. Tissue burning to stop bleeding.
2. Light beam-based cutting method.
3. Gripping instrument for tissues.
7. Surgical thread for wound closure.

Solution on page 100

PUZZLE 33
HUMAN ANATOMY

Medical Generalities and Miscellaneous

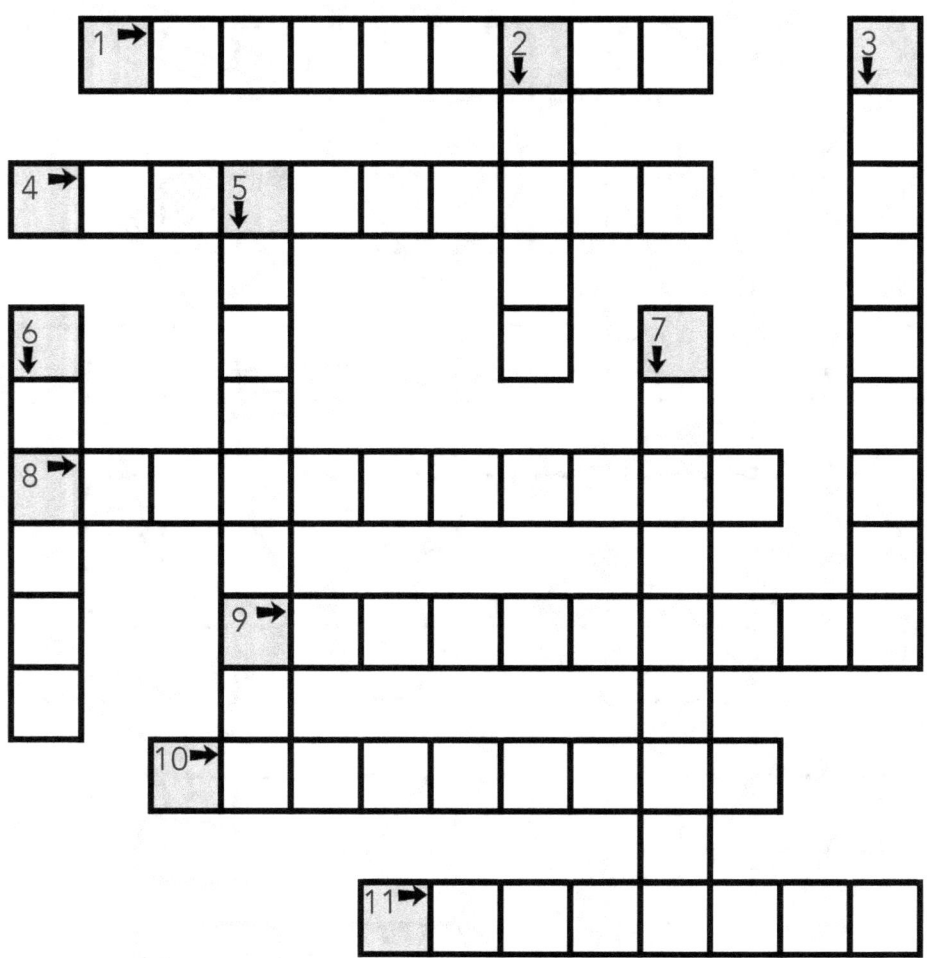

ACROSS

1. Respiratory muscle separating thorax and abdomen.
4. Tissue producing blood cells.
8. System transporting blood throughout body.
9. Digestive organs absorbing nutrients.
10. Spinal column bones protecting spinal cord.
11. Body's supportive and protective framework.

DOWN

2. Largest artery carrying oxygenated blood.
3. Outermost layer of skin.
5. Hormone-secreting gland system.
6. Upper arm muscle flexing elbow.
7. Flexible connective tissue in joints.

Solution on page 100

PUZZLE 34
ENVIRONMENTAL HEALTH

Medical Generalities and Miscellaneous

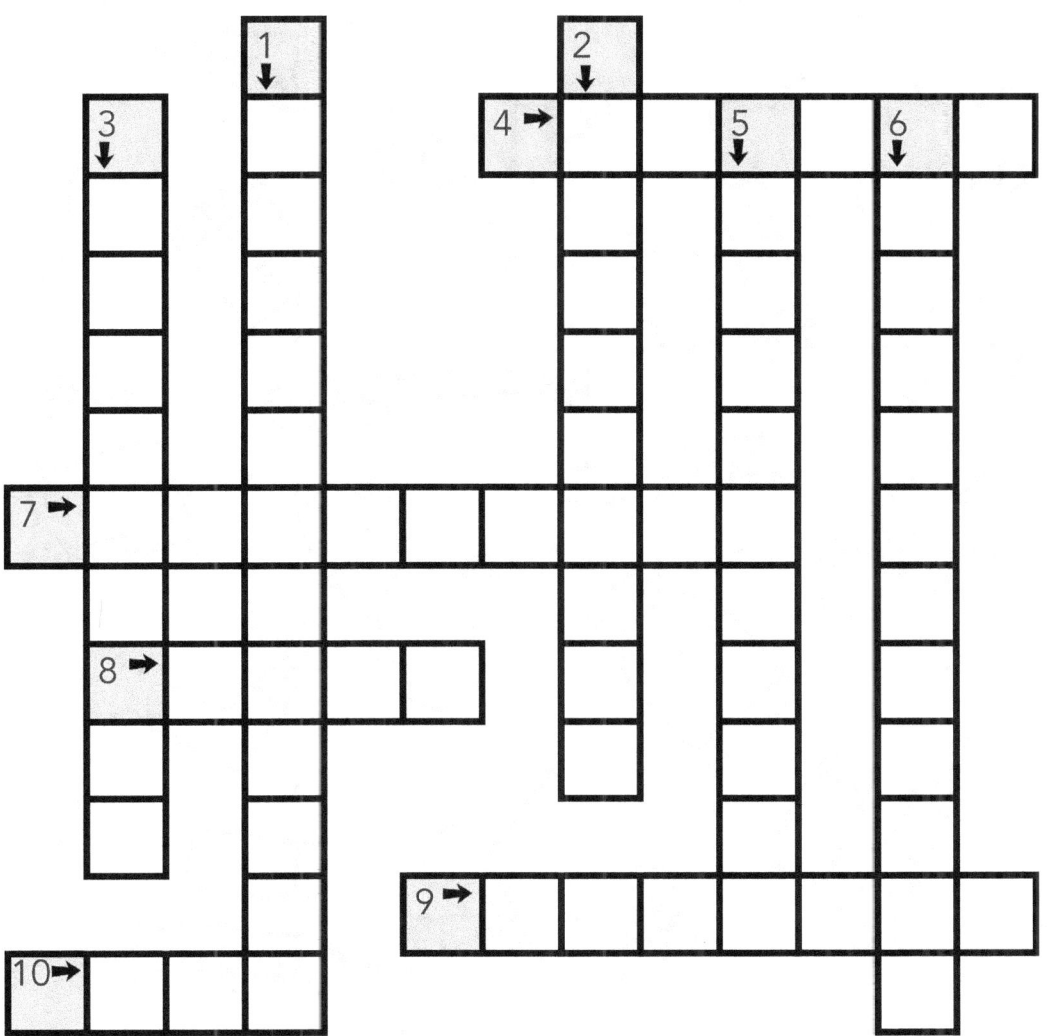

ACROSS

4. Neurotoxic element in thermometers and seafood.
7. Hygienic practices preventing disease spread.
8. Fecal coliform bacteria in contaminated water.
9. Fibrous mineral causing lung diseases.
10. Air pollution reducing urban visibility.

DOWN

1. Heavy metal toxicity from paint.
2. Chemicals controlling agricultural pests.
3. Preventing foodborne illness outbreaks.
5. Cancer-causing environmental agents.
6. Silent Spring author, environmentalist pioneer.

PUZZLE 35
NUTRITION AND DIETETICS

Medical Generalities and Miscellaneous

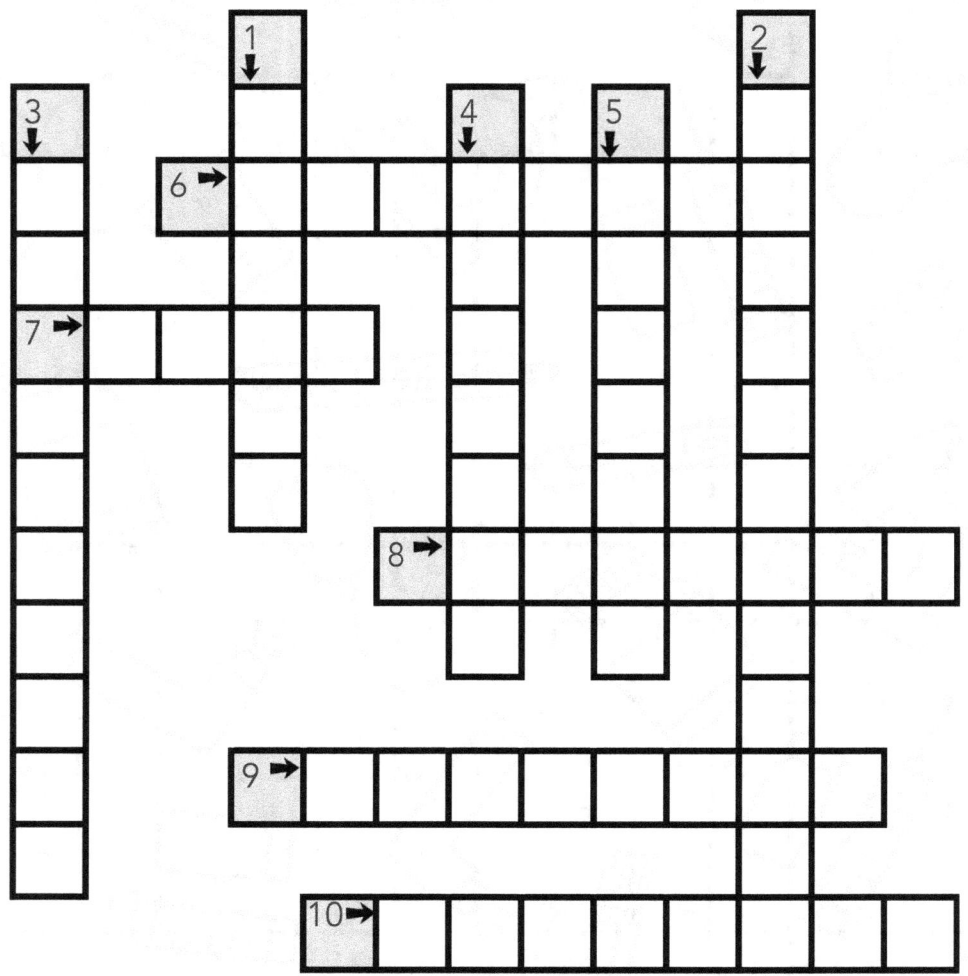

ACROSS

6. Nutrient-enhanced food production process.
7. Indigestible plant matter aiding digestion.
8. Advance culinary organization technique.
9. Nutritional information packaging requirement.
10. High-fat, low-carbohydrate dietary approach.

DOWN

1. Essential macronutrient for tissue repair.
2. Heart-healthy eating pattern from region.
3. Nutrient-dense vegetable category.
4. Blood glucose regulation disorder.
5. Inorganic nutrients for bodily functions.

Solution on page 100

PUZZLE 36
WOMEN'S HEALTH

Medical Generalities and Miscellaneous

ACROSS

2. Pioneer of family planning clinics.
4. Transitional phase before menopause onset.
5. Monthly uterine lining shedding process.
6. Gestation period of fetal development.
7. Breast tissue X-ray screening procedure.
8. Cervical cancer prevention immunization.
9. Contraceptive methods for family planning.

DOWN

1. Cervical cell screening examination.
3. Malignant neoplasm of female gonads.

Solution on page 100

41

PUZZLE 37
ALTERNATIVE MEDICINE

Medical Generalities and Miscellaneous

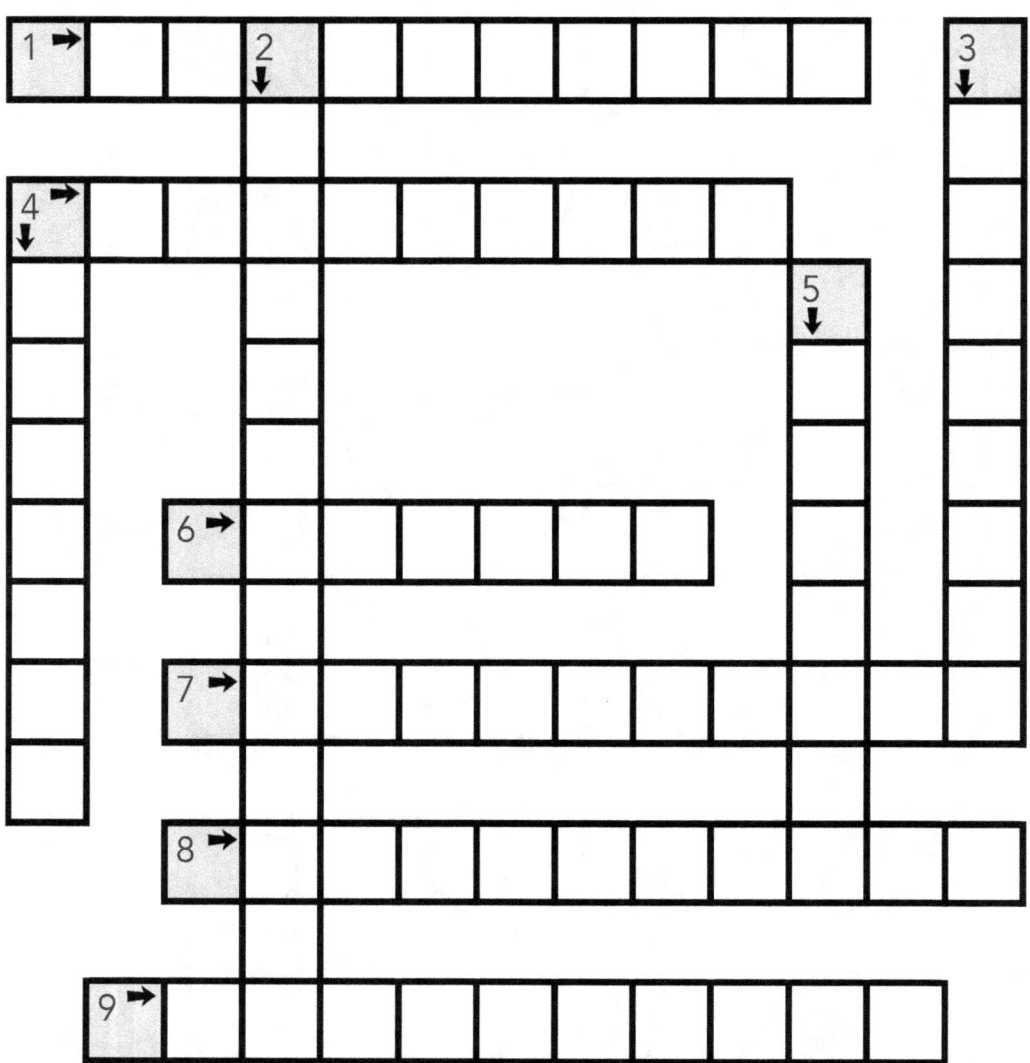

ACROSS

1. Study of body movement mechanics.
4. Diluted substance treatment approach.
6. Energy centers in subtle body.
7. Floral essence emotional remedies.
8. Physiological self-regulation technique.
9. Posture-based healing practice.

DOWN

2. Non-contact biofield manipulation.
3. Vital energy pathways in body.
4. Whole-person health consideration.
5. Ancient Indian wellness system.

Solution on page 100

PUZZLE 38
PARASITES

Medical Generalities and Miscellaneous

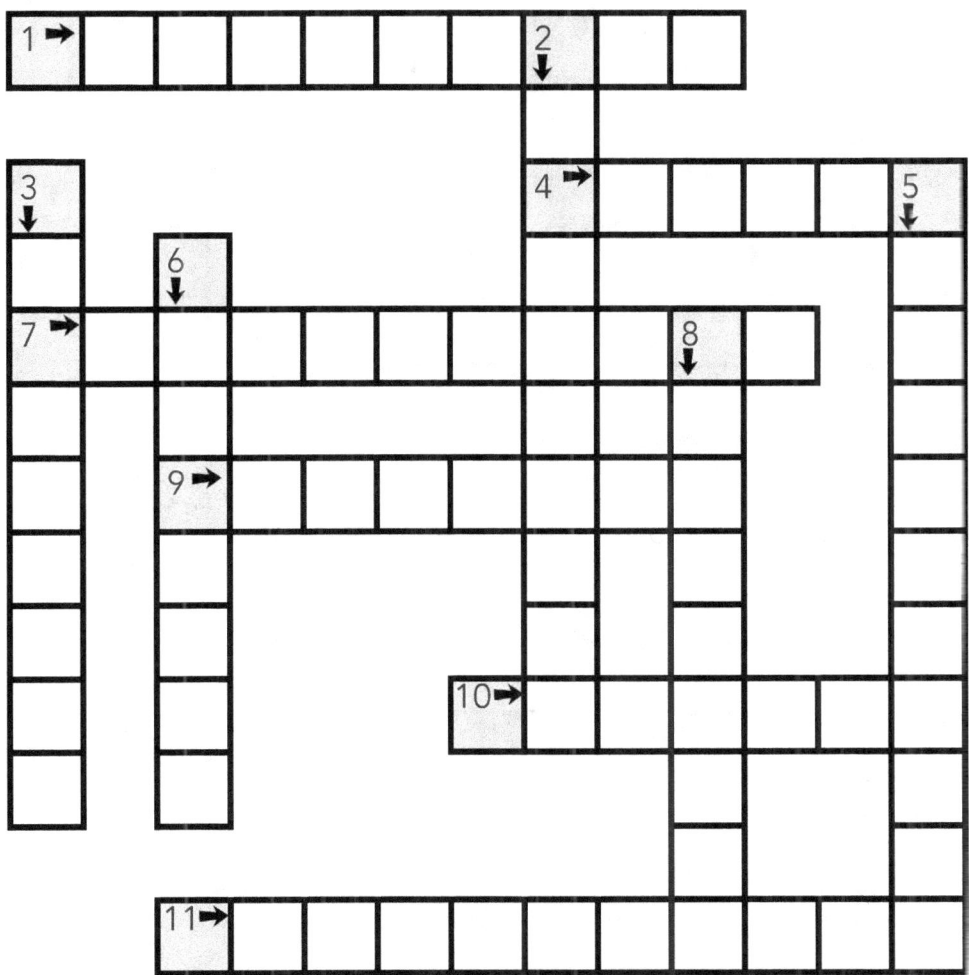

ACROSS

1. Intestinal infection caused by Giardia lamblia.
4. Resistant stage in coccidian lifecycle.
7. Active feeding stage of protozoan parasite.
9. Roundworm with cylindrical unsegmented body.
10. Tapeworm with segmented body structure.
11. Presence of parasites in bloodstream.

DOWN

2. Infective stage of malaria parasite.
3. Genus of amoeboid protozoan parasites.
5. Genus causing trichinosis in humans.
6. Disease transmitted from animals to humans.
8. Parasitic flatworm with leaf-like body.

Solution on page 100

43

PUZZLE 39
EXPLORING TOXICOLOGY

Medical Generalities and Miscellaneous

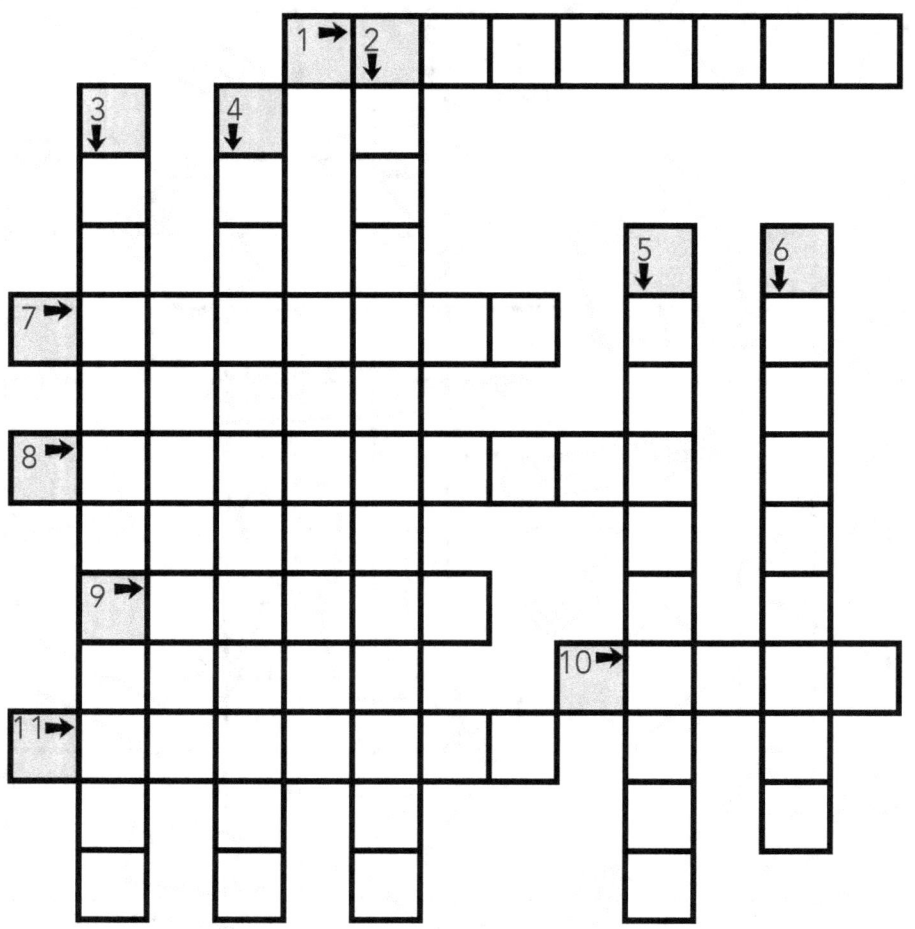

ACROSS

1. Developmental toxin affecting fetal growth.
7. Toxin-producing organism's defense mechanism.
8. Foreign substance metabolized by organism.
9. Substance causing injury or death.
10. Biologically produced poisonous compound.
11. Substance counteracting effects of poison.

DOWN

2. Study of pollutants' effects on ecosystems.
3. Relationship between exposure and effect.
4. Damage to genetic material by toxins.
5. Cancer-causing substance or agent.
6. Process removing heavy metals from body.

Solution on page 100

PUZZLE 40
BIOCHEMICAL PATHWAYS

Medical Generalities and Miscellaneous

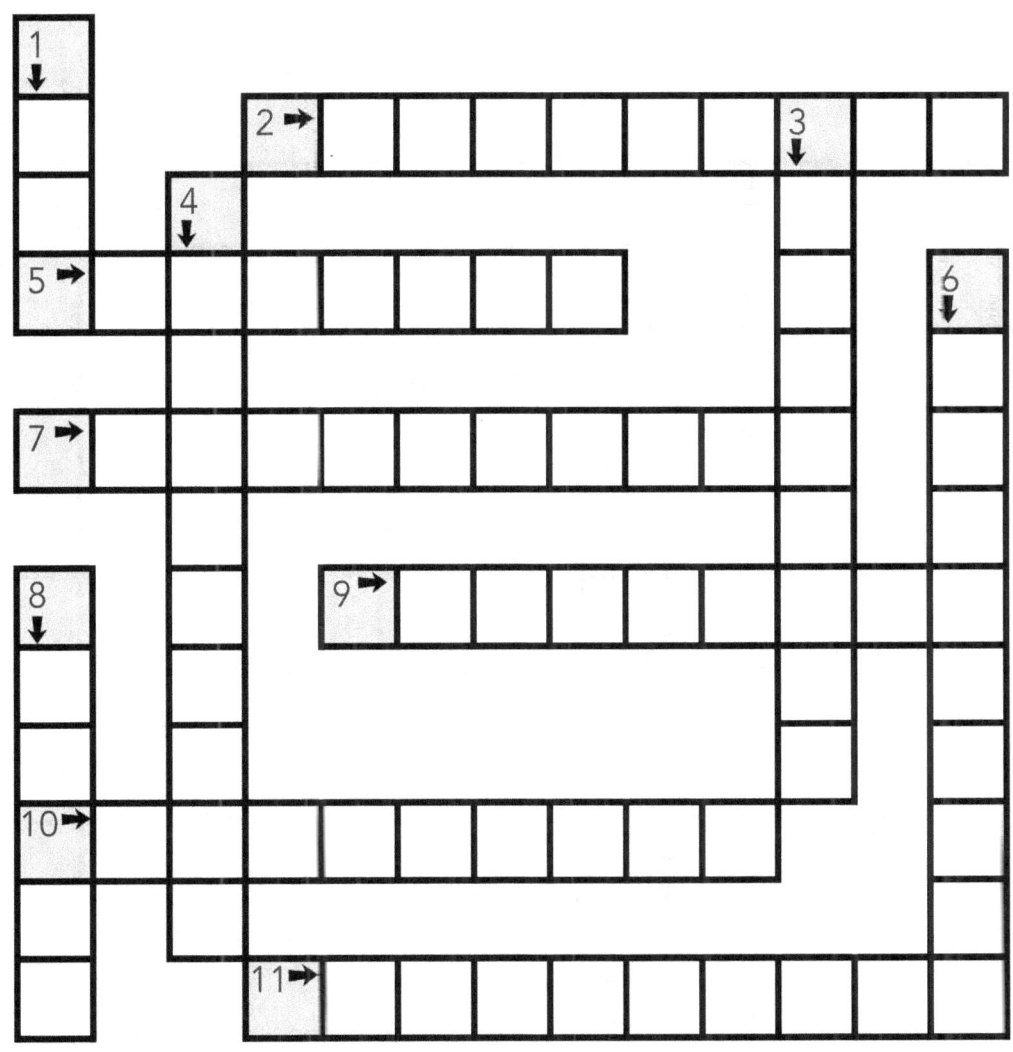

ACROSS
2. Protein regulation via non-active site binding.
5. Enzyme unwinding DNA double helix.
7. Building blocks of nucleic acids.
9. Non-protein enzyme cofactors.
10. Protein building block monomers.
11. Enzyme's substrate-binding region.

DOWN
1. Reduced form of nicotinamide adenine dinucleotide.
3. Cellular protein synthesis factories.
4. Glucose breakdown pathway.
6. Citric acid cycle of metabolism.
8. Enzyme catalyzing molecular bond formation.

Solution on page 101

PUZZLE 41
MEDICAL ETHICS

Medical Generalities and Miscellaneous

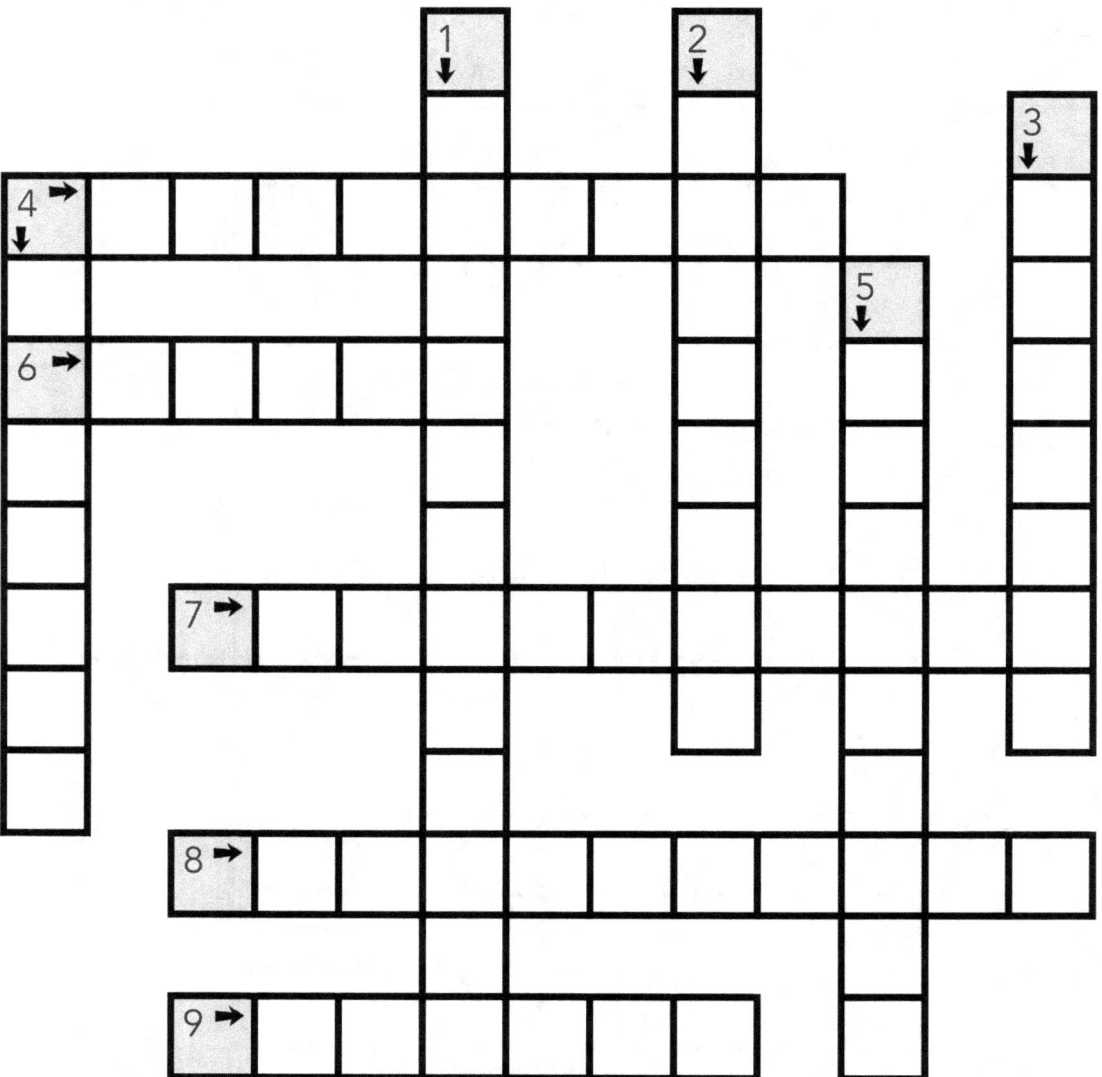

ACROSS
4. Resource distribution in healthcare systems.
6. Patient prioritization in emergencies.
7. Principle of doing good.
8. Altering DNA sequences.
9. Fairness in healthcare access.

DOWN
1. Perceived benefit without treatment.
2. Moral implications of medical advances.
3. No resuscitation directive.
4. Patient self-determination in care.
5. Advanced healthcare directive document.

Solution on page 101

PUZZLE 42
PHARMACOLOGY

Medical Generalities and Miscellaneous

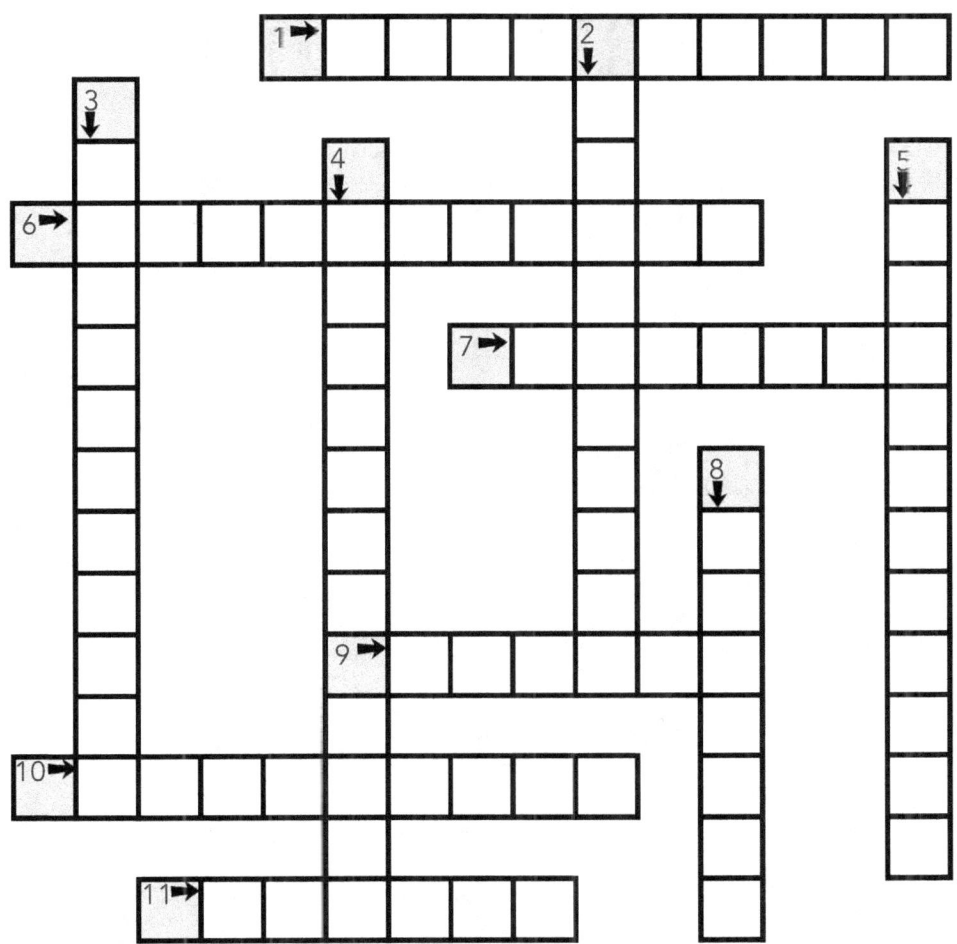

ACROSS

1. Unapproved pharmaceutical application.
6. Multiple medication use in patient.
7. Drug elimination time measurement.
9. Biologically inactive pharmaceutical precursor.
10. Receptor-blocking compound.
11. Common analgesic and antipyretic medication.

DOWN

2. Adrenergic receptor-inhibiting cardiovascular drug.
3. Cholesterol-lowering HMG-CoA reductase inhibitor.
4. Essential structural features for bioactivity.
5. Medication effect vs. concentration relationship.
8. Pharmaceutical compound interactions.

Solution on page 101

PUZZLE 43
BACTERIOLOGY

Medical Generalities and Miscellaneous

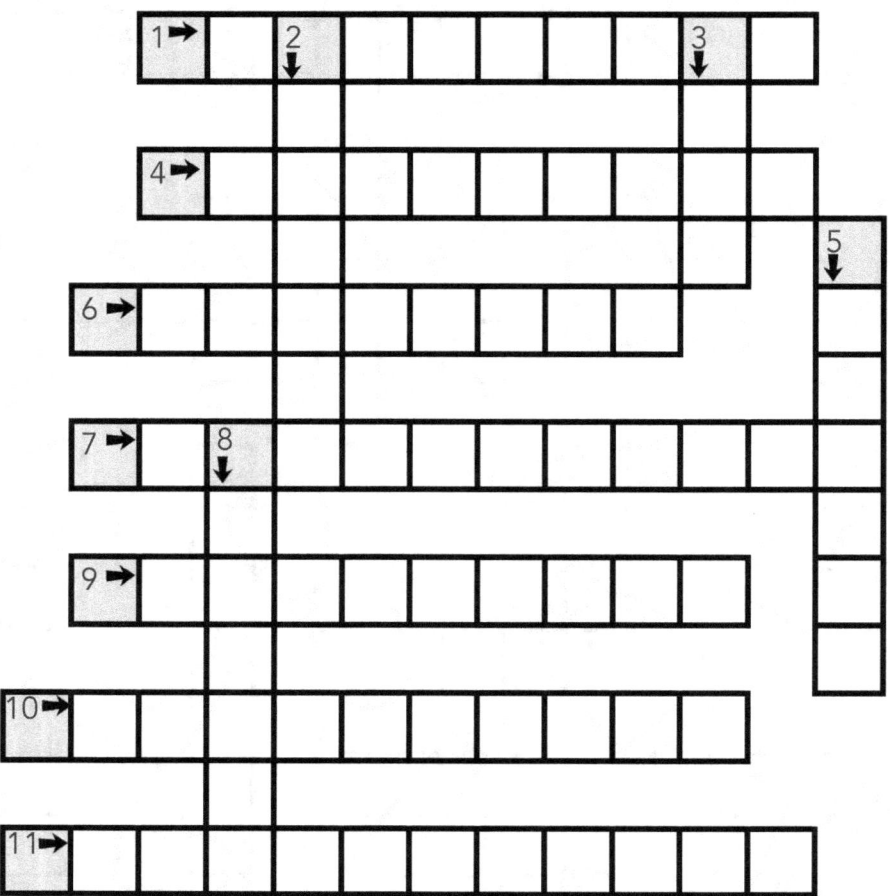

ACROSS

1. Technique for visualizing bacterial structures.
4. Genus causing foodborne gastroenteritis.
6. Inflammatory lung condition from microorganisms.
7. Infectious disease caused by Mycobacterium.
9. Beneficial microorganisms for gut health.
10. Test determining bacterial antibiotic sensitivity.
11. Bacterial classification using dye retention.

DOWN

2. Method for growing microorganisms in lab.
3. Hair-like bacterial surface appendages.
5. Extrachromosomal DNA in bacterial cells.
8. Microbial community adhering to surfaces.

Solution on page 101

PUZZLE 44
EMERGENCY PRESCRIPTIONS

Medical Generalities and Miscellaneous

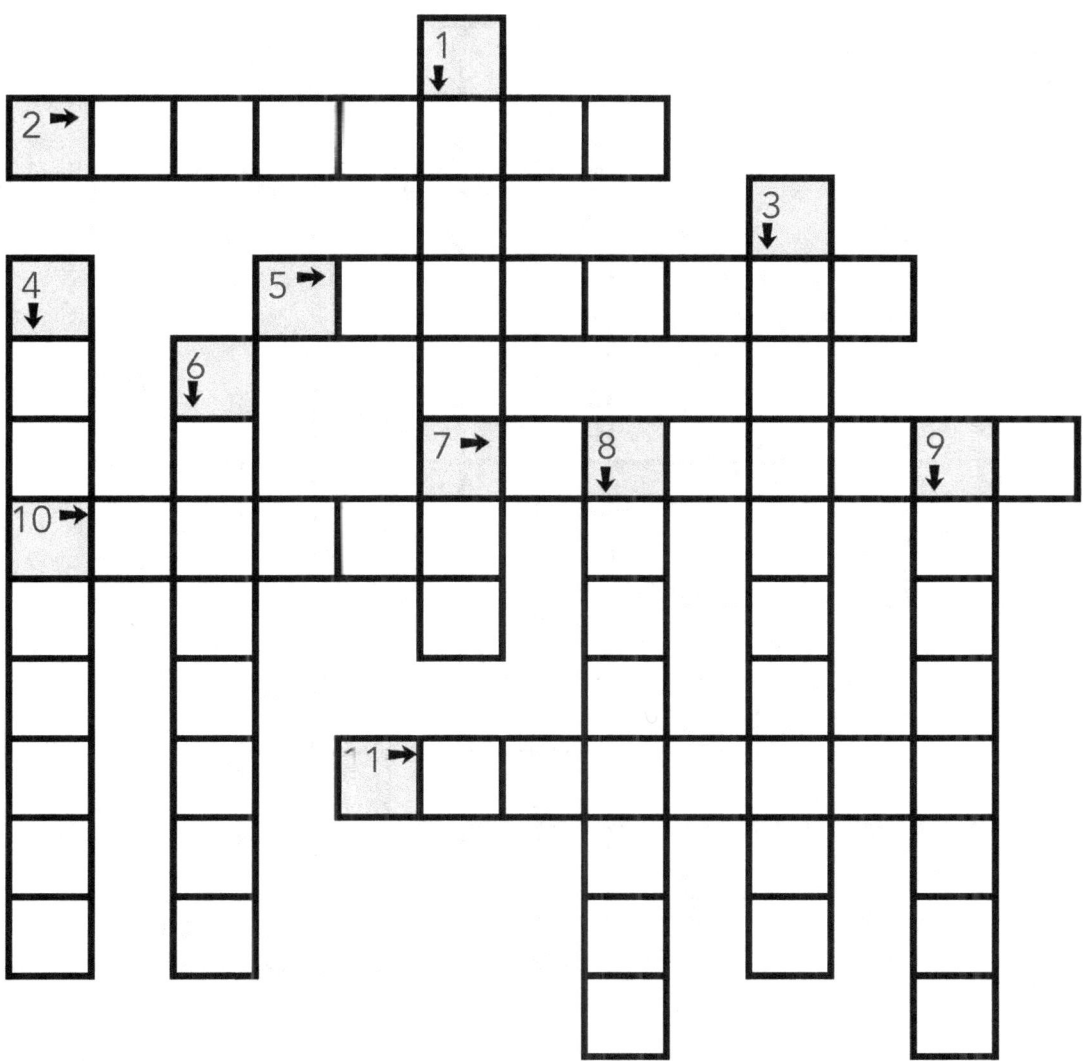

ACROSS
2. Cardiac contractility enhancer.
5. Neurotransmitter used for shock.
7. Parenteral hydration solutions.
10. Opioid overdose reversal agent.
11. Dissociative anesthetic for sedation.

4. Supraventricular tachycardia treatment.
6. Anticholinergic for bracycardia.
8. Synthetic opioid analgesic.
9. Medication promoting urine output.

DOWN
1. Potent opioid pain reliever.
3. Airway management procedure.

PUZZLE 45
FUNGAL BIOLOGY

Medical Generalities and Miscellaneous

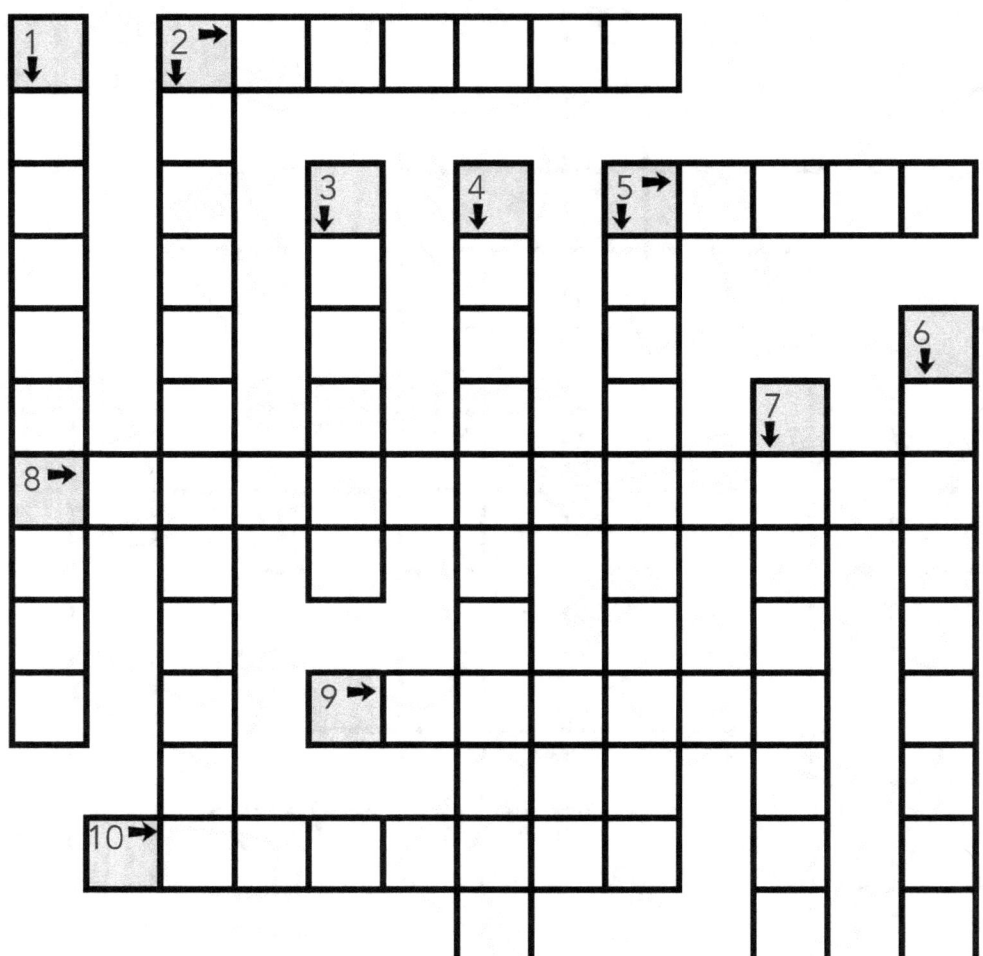

ACROSS

2. Discoverer of penicillin from Penicillium mold.
5. Reproductive unit of fungi.
8. Unwanted microbial growth in culture.
9. Genus containing deadly poisonous mushrooms.
10. Vegetative part of fungal organism.

DOWN

1. Technique for observing minute fungal structures.
2. Reproductive structure of macroscopic fungi.
3. Filamentous growth units of fungi.
4. Yeast infection caused by Candida species.
5. Structure containing asexual fungal spores.
6. Chemical agent that kills fungi.
7. Taxonomist who classified fungi as plants.

Solution on page 101

PUZZLE 46
LAB DIAGNOSTICS

Medical Generalities and Miscellaneous

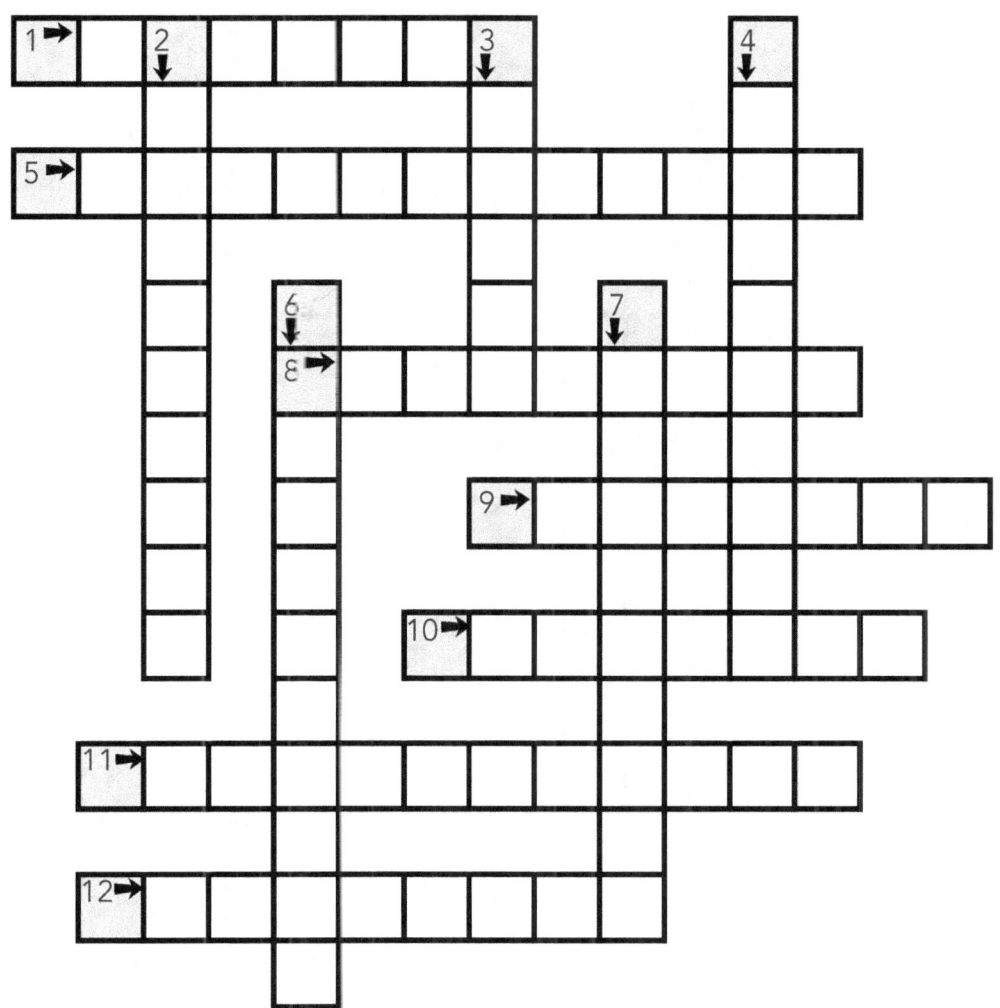

ACROSS
1. Blood cancer affecting white cells.
5. Lipid measured in lipid panel.
8. Liver inflammation diagnostic markers.
9. Iron storage protein blood test.
10. Cervical cancer screening procedure.
11. Mycobacterium detection in sputum.
12. ABO and Rh factor test.

DOWN
2. Urine composition diagnostic examination.
3. Hemoglobin deficiency screening test.
4. Kidney function indicator in serum.
6. Lipid panel cardiovascular risk marker.
7. Cellular examination magnification instrument.

Solution on page 101

PUZZLE 47
PEDIATRIC PATHOLOGIES

Medical Generalities and Miscellaneous

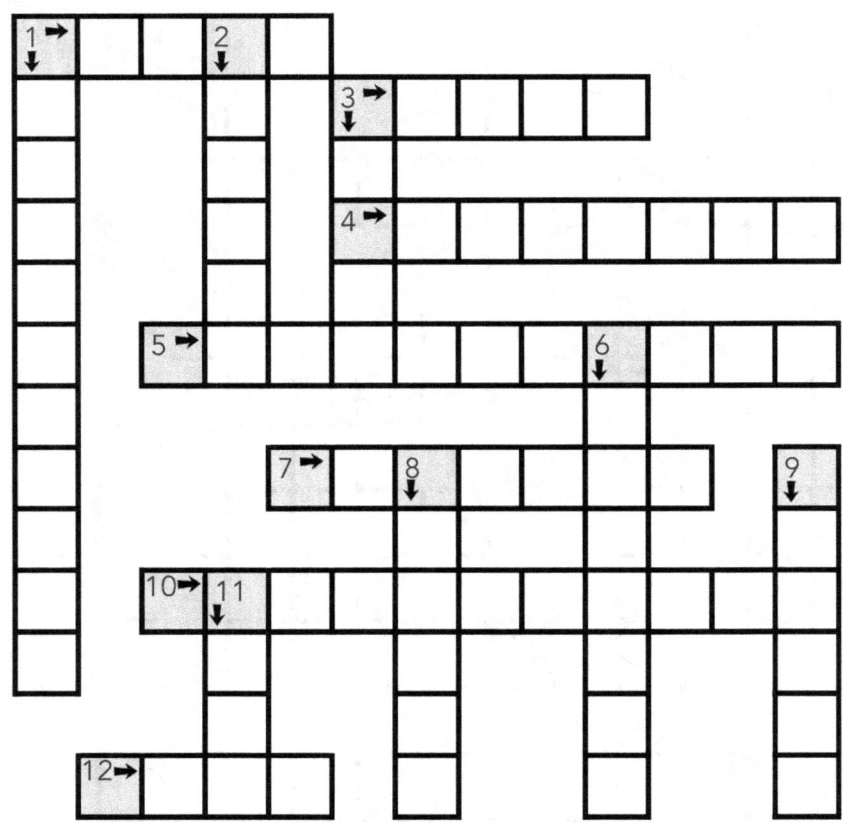

ACROSS

1. Elevated body temperature symptom.
3. Respiratory infection with barking cough.
4. Cancer of blood-forming tissues.
5. Preventive inoculation against diseases.
7. Highly contagious viral exanthematous disease.
10. Tool tracking pediatric development.
12. Neurodevelopmental disorder affecting attention span.

DOWN

1. Immune response to specific edibles.
2. Inflammatory skin condition causing itching.
3. Prolonged crying in seemingly healthy infants.
6. Process of tooth eruption in infants.
8. Chronic respiratory condition with airway inflammation.
9. Neurodevelopmental disorder affecting social interaction.
11. Skin eruption indicating various conditions.

Solution on page 102

PUZZLE 48
VIROLOGY BASICS

Medical Generalities and Miscellaneous

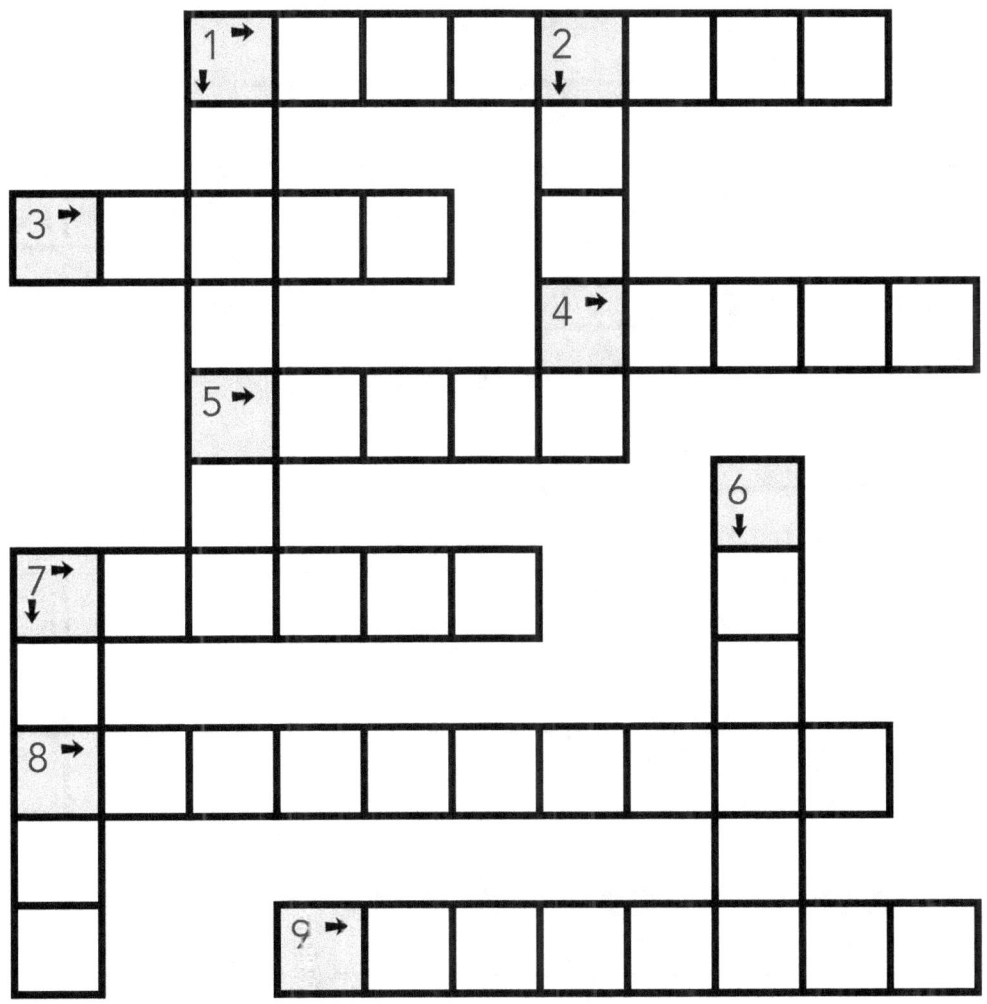

ACROSS
1. Global disease outbreak.
3. Cell membrane destruction process.
4. Bacteriophage research pioneer.
5. Antibody detection laboratory technique.
7. Complete virus particle.
8. Antiviral nucleotide analog drug.
9. Animal-to-human disease transmission.

DOWN
1. Vaccine development pioneer.
2. Hemorrhagic fever-causing filovirus.
6. Neurotropic lyssavirus infection.
7. Non-living infectious genetic agent.

Solution on page 102

PUZZLE 49
ENTOMOLOGICAL DISEASES

Medical Generalities and Miscellaneous

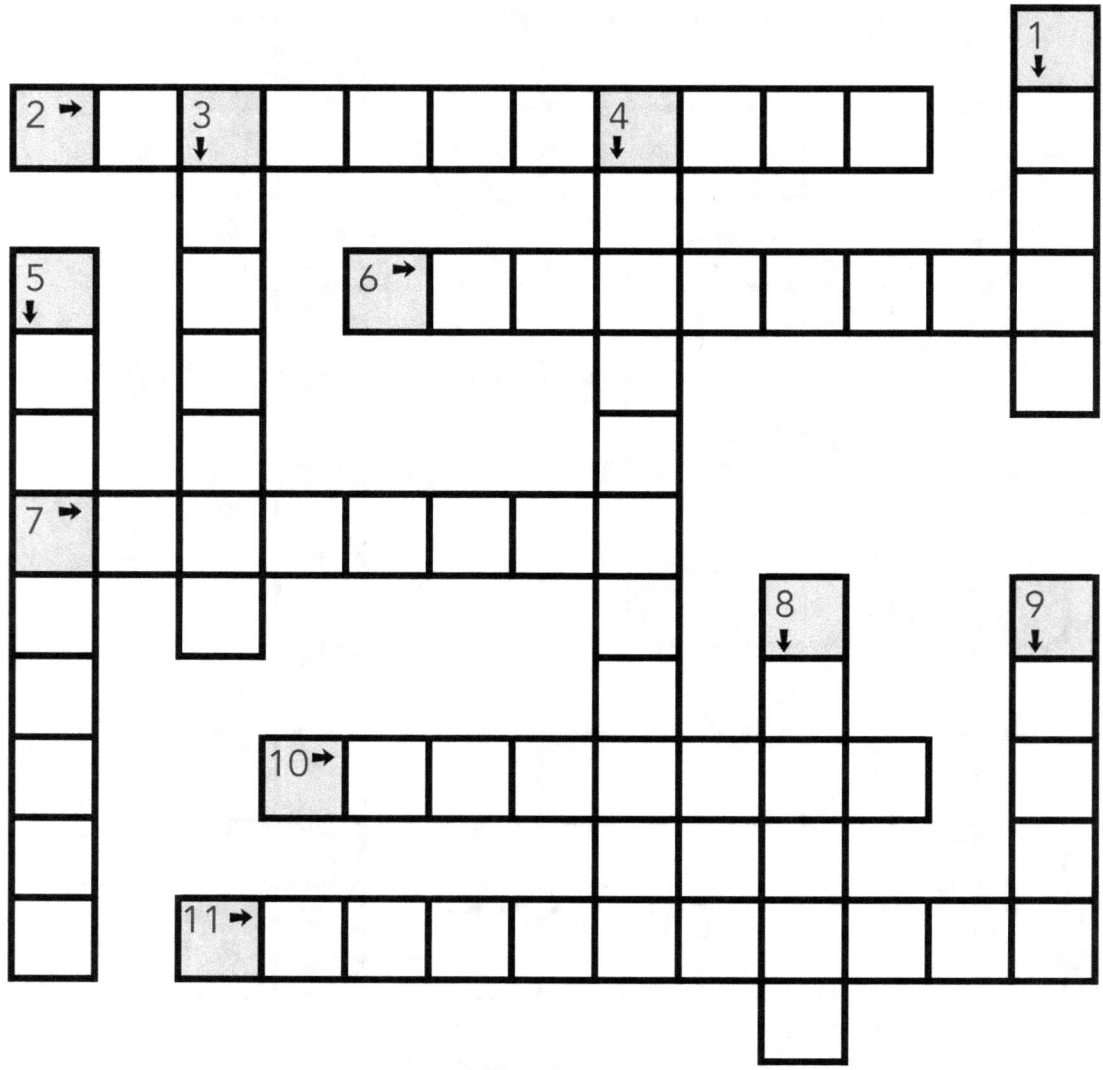

ACROSS

2. Tick-borne spirochetal infection.
6. Rabbit fever bacterial disease.
7. Widespread outbreak of disease.
10. Region prone to vector-borne illnesses.
11. Mosquito-transmitted viral arthritis.

3. Mosquito-borne parasitic fever.
4. Complete elimination of disease.
5. Substance deterring insect vectors.
8. Flea-transmitted bacterial infection.
9. Fruit bat-associated hemorrhagic fever.

DOWN

1. Insect vectors of bubonic plague.

Solution on page 102

PUZZLE 50
FAMOUS MEDICAL JOURNALS

Medical Generalities and Miscellaneous

ACROSS
5. British medical journal's abbreviation.
7. Researcher's impact metric.
9. Free scientific literature availability.
11. Australian medical journal's acronym.
12. Prominent British medical periodical.
3. Top US medical journal.
4. Infectious disease expert's surname.
6. Brain disorders medical specialty.
8. American Medical Association's publication.
10. Leading journal in biology

DOWN
1. Biomedical research funding platform.
2. Free full-text archive database.

Solution on page 102

55

PUZZLE 51
A SWEET BUT DANGEROUS CONDITION

Clinical Cases

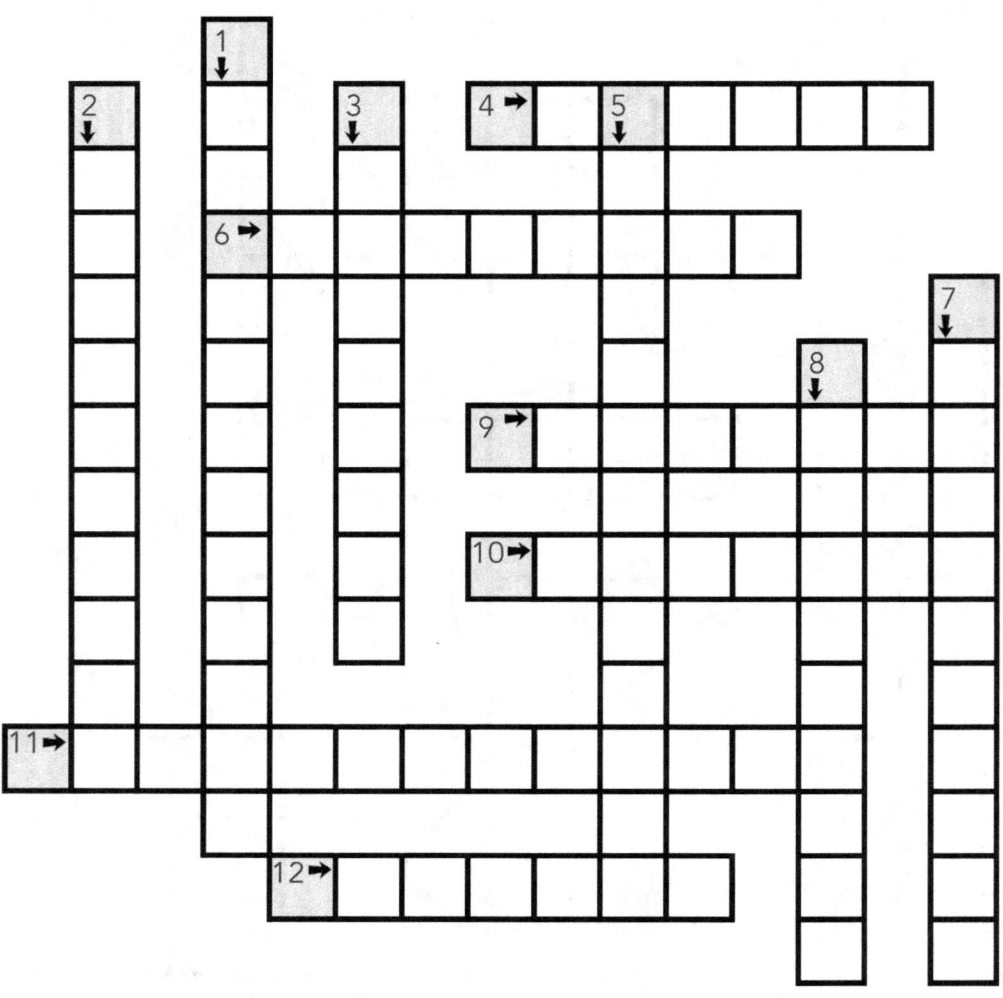

ACROSS
4. Hormone regulating blood sugar levels.
6. Endocrine cells producing key hormone.
9. Organ secreting digestive enzymes.
10. Excessive urination condition.
11. Elevated blood sugar state.
12. Primary monosaccharide in blood.

DOWN
1. Macronutrients broken down into sugars.
2. Kidney damage from chronic condition.
3. First-line medication for metabolic disorder.
5. Drugs stimulating insulin secretion.
7. Occurring during pregnancy.
8. Nerve damage from metabolic imbalance.

Solution on page 102

PUZZLE 52
THE SILENT PRESSURE WITHIN

Clinical Cases

ACROSS
2. Myocardial infarction due to blocked arteries.
4. Medications promoting fluid excretion.
8. Abnormal protein presence in urine.
9. Enzyme regulating blood pressure homeostasis.
10. Eating plan for cardiovascular health.

DOWN
1. Damage to retinal blood vessels.
3. Steroid hormone affecting sodium retention.
5. Upper number in blood pressure reading.
6. Cerebrovascular event probability factor.
7. Lower number in blood pressure reading.

Solution on page 102

PUZZLE 53
BREATHLESS IN THE NIGHT

Clinical Cases

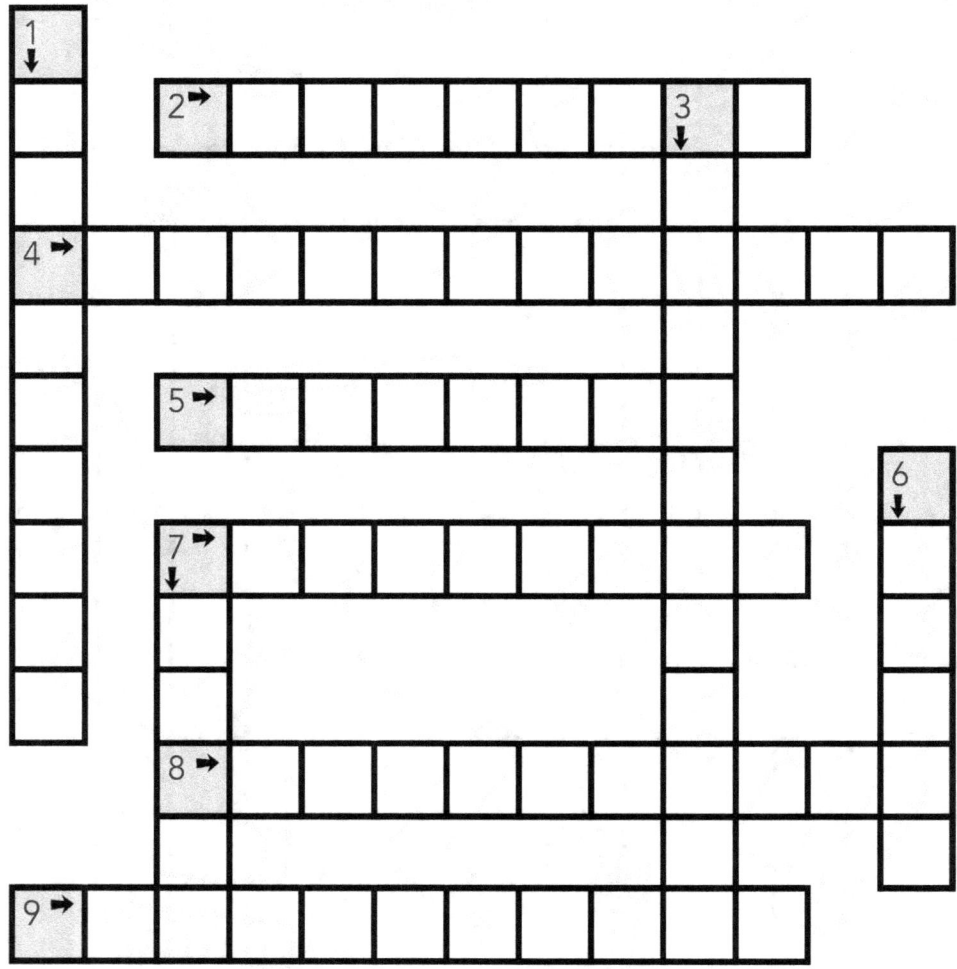

ACROSS

2. Bronchodilator medication for airway constriction.
4. Emergency breathing aid device.
5. Respiratory medication delivery devices.
7. Allergenic animal skin particles.
8. Inflammatory mediator in immune responses.
9. Oral medication for bronchial inflammation.

DOWN

1. Lung function measurement test.
3. Systemic anti-inflammatory medications.
6. Inhaler attachment for improved delivery.
7. Allergenic plant reproductive particles.

Solution on page 102

PUZZLE 54
A BREATHLESS BATTLE

Clinical Cases

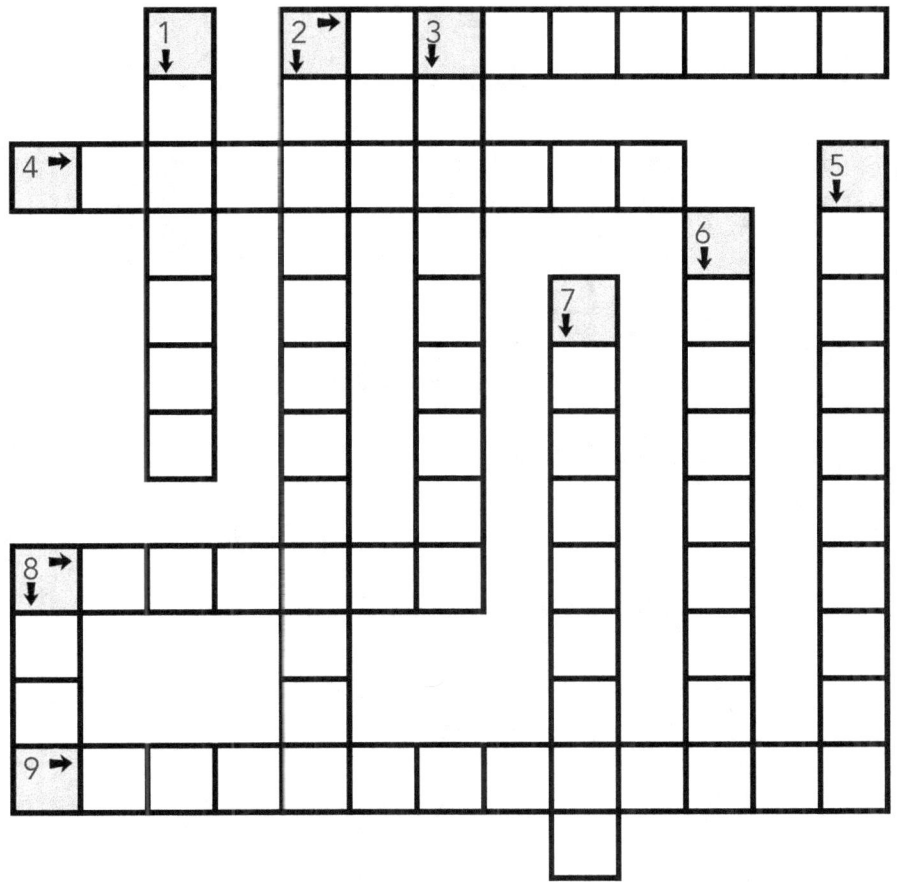

ACROSS

2. Imaging technique for thoracic visualization.
4. Long-acting anticholinergic bronchodilator medication.
8. Subjective sensation of breathing difficulty.
9. Supplemental O2 administration for hypoxemia.

DOWN

1. Major risk factor for respiratory diseases.
2. Right ventricular enlargement from pulmonary hypertension.
3. Alveolar wall destruction and hyperinflation.
5. Pulmonary function test measuring airflow.
6. Lung infection causing alveolar inflammation.
7. Device delivering aerosolized medication therapeutically.
8. Pulmonary gas exchange capacity measurement.

Solution on page 102

PUZZLE 55
WHEN THE HEART'S PATHWAYS ARE BLOCKED

Clinical Cases

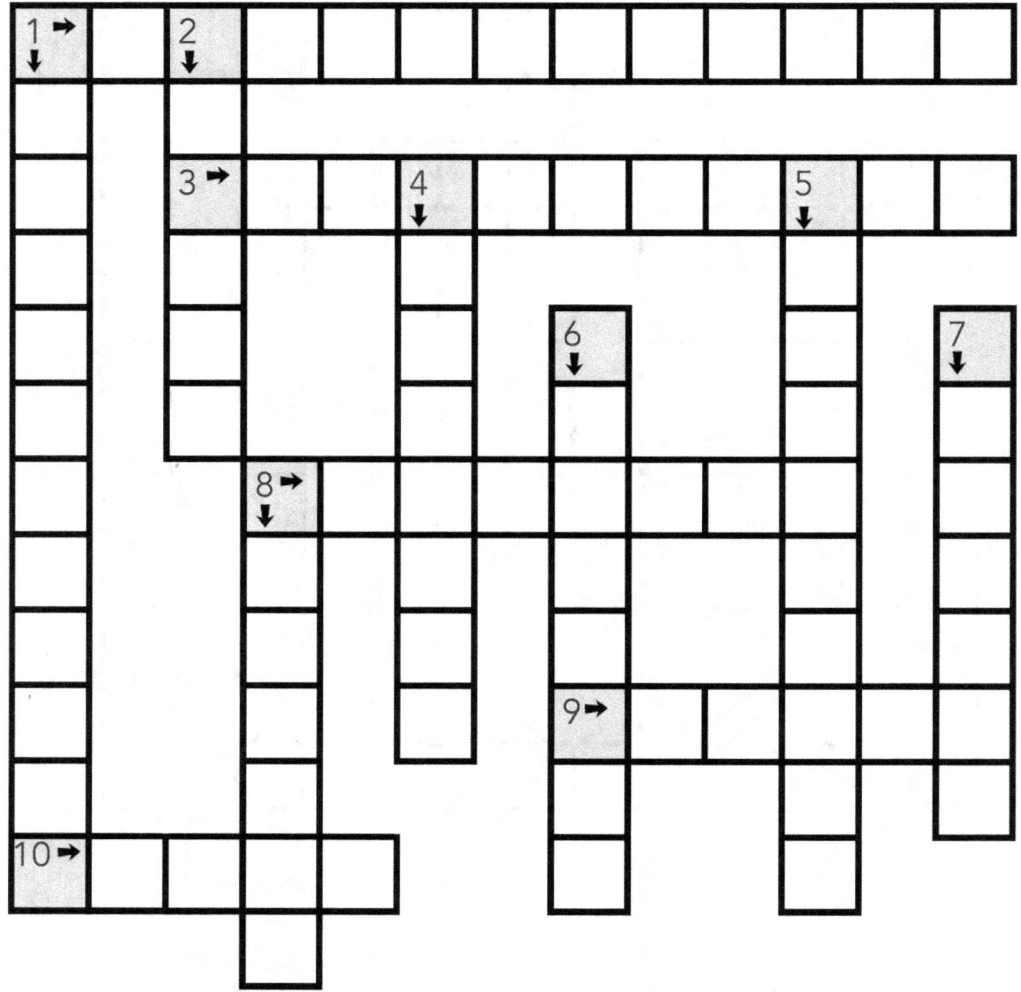

ACROSS
1. Rerouting blood flow around blockage.
3. Widening narrowed blood vessels.
8. Abnormal narrowing of blood vessels.
9. Partial heart muscle damage event.
10. Tubular support for blood vessels.
4. Inadequate blood supply to tissues.
5. Cardiac function assessment procedure.
6. Protein indicating heart muscle damage.
7. Blood-thinning pain relief medication.
8. Cholesterol-lowering pharmaceutical agents.

DOWN
1. Heart rate lowering medications.
2. Fatty deposits in artery walls.

Solution on page 103

PUZZLE 56
A SUDDEN LOSS OF CONNECTION

Clinical Cases

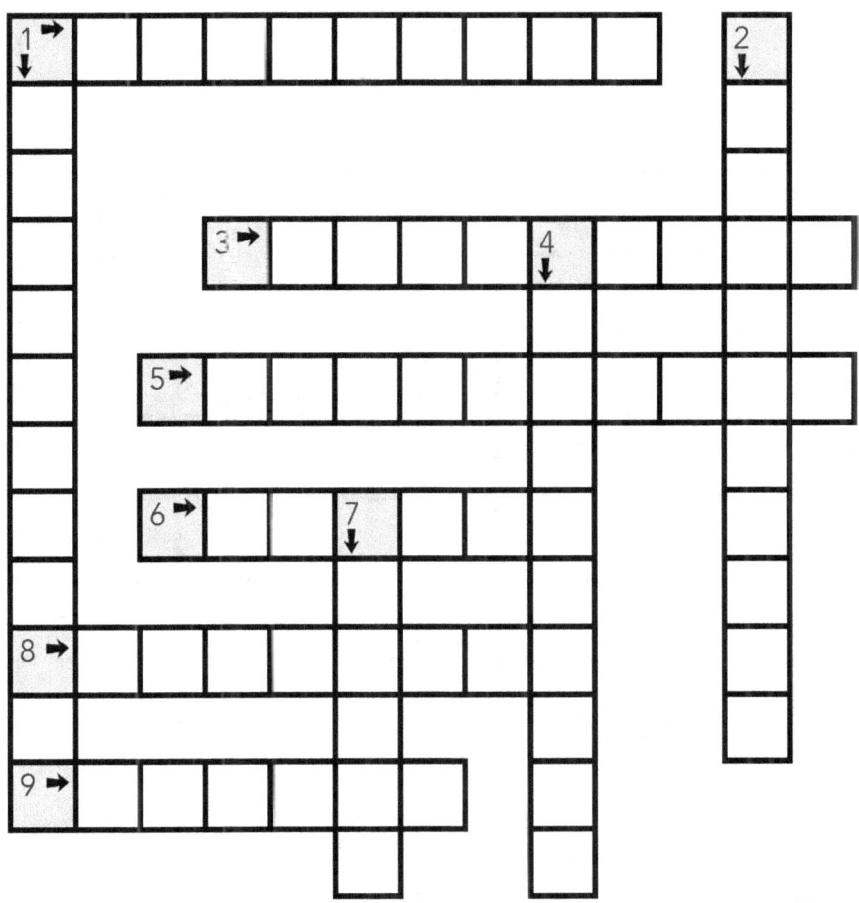

ACROSS
1. Impaired articulation due to neurological dysfunction.
3. Related to blood clot formation.
5. Imaging technique visualizing blood vessels.
6. Language impairment following brain injury.
8. Difficulty swallowing due to neuromuscular disorder.
9. Pertaining to circulating material obstructing vessels.

DOWN
1. Time metric in emergency medical treatment.
2. Weakness affecting one side of body.
4. Brain region crucial for speech production.
7. Impaired coordination of voluntary movements.

Solution on page 103

PUZZLE 57
A JOINT AFFAIR

Clinical Cases

ACROSS
5. Destruction of osseous tissue.
6. Joint lining membrane inflammation.
7. Tissue response to injury.
9. Antimetabolite used in chemotherapy.
11. Sudden worsening of symptoms.
12. Period of symptom reduction.

DOWN
1. Flexible connective tissue.
2. Abnormal tissue growth.
3. Alteration in body structure.
4. Self-directed immune system attack.
8. Persistent feeling of exhaustion.
10. Diagnostic imaging using radiation.

Solution on page 103

PUZZLE 58
A SLOW DECLINE IN FUNCTION

Clinical Cases

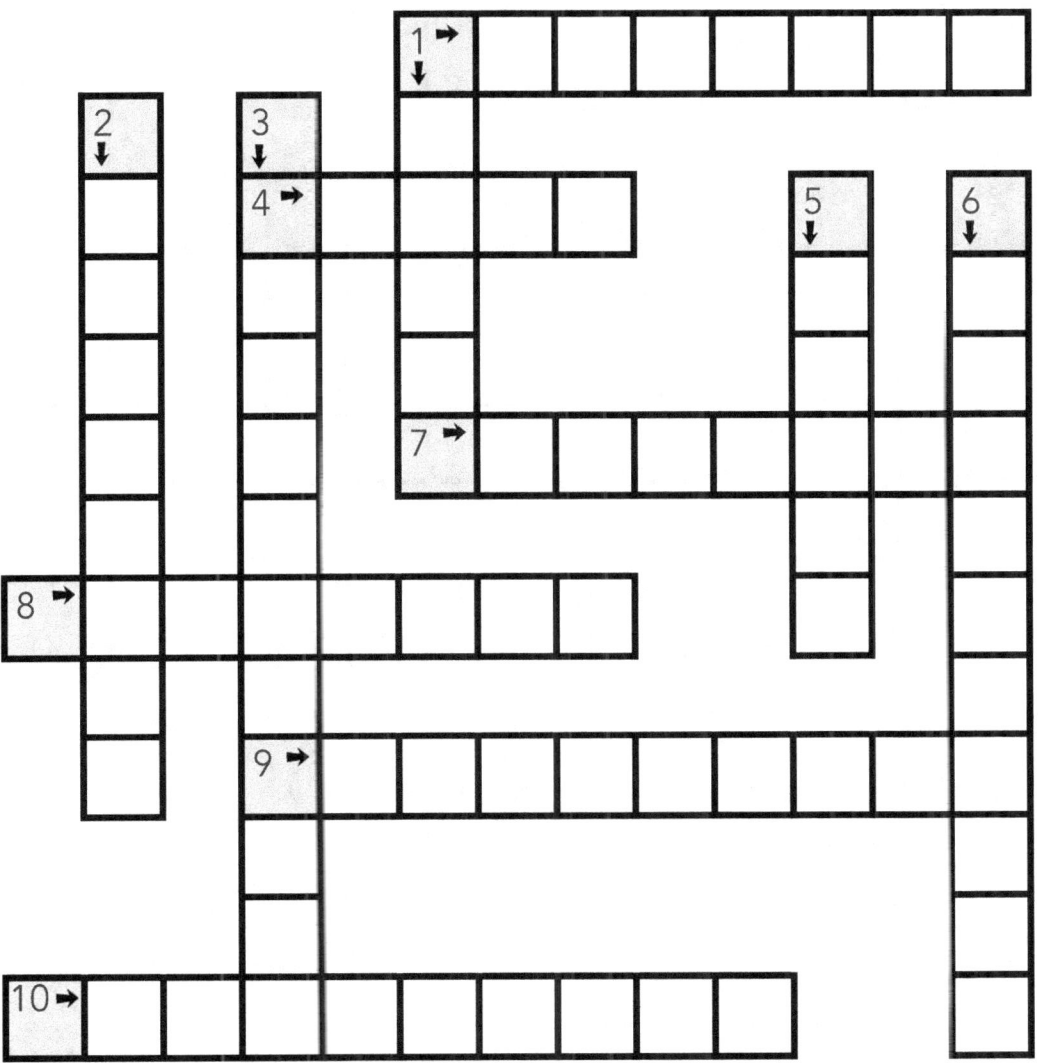

ACROSS

1. Excess acid accumulation in bodily fluids.
4. Abnormal fluid retention in tissues.
7. Elevated nitrogenous compounds in blood.
8. Blood purification process.
9. Relating to kidney filtering units.
10. Removal of waste from blood.

DOWN

1. Reduced red blood cell count.
2. Medications promoting urine production.
3. Kidney disease specialist.
5. Waste product buildup in blood.
6. Calcium-regulating endocrine glands.

Solution on page 103

PUZZLE 59
BONES OF GLASS

Clinical Cases

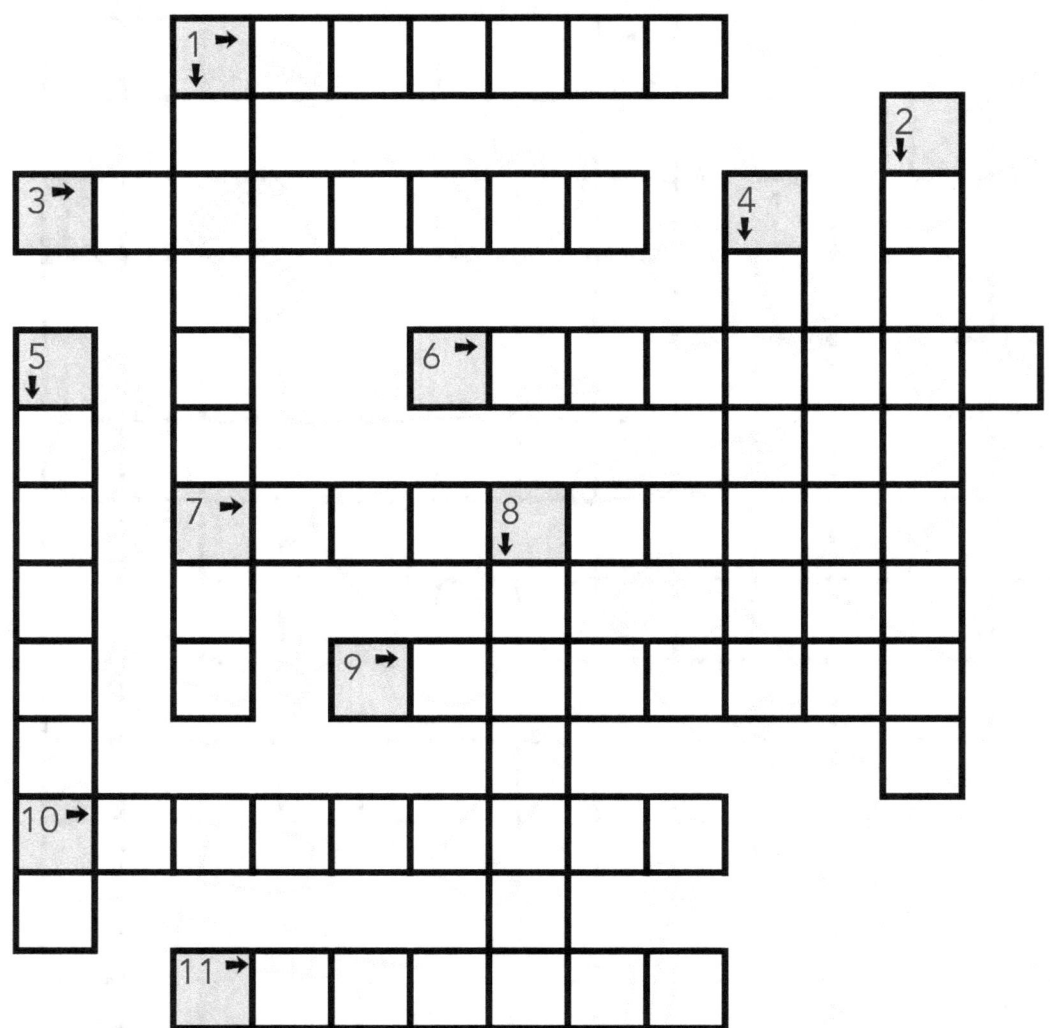

ACROSS
1. Measure of bone mineral content.
3. Study of hereditary factors in disease.
6. Key hormone in bone metabolism.
7. Prescribed treatment for bone health.
9. Protein crucial for bone structure.
10. Dietary factors affecting bone health.
11. Bisphosphonate drug for bone treatment.

DOWN
1. Monoclonal antibody for bone therapy.
2. Diagnostic test for bone health.
4. Habit impacting bone mineral density.
5. Nutrient essential for calcium absorption.
8. Mineral vital for bone strength.

Solution on page 103

PUZZLE 60
THE MEMORY THIEF

Clinical Cases

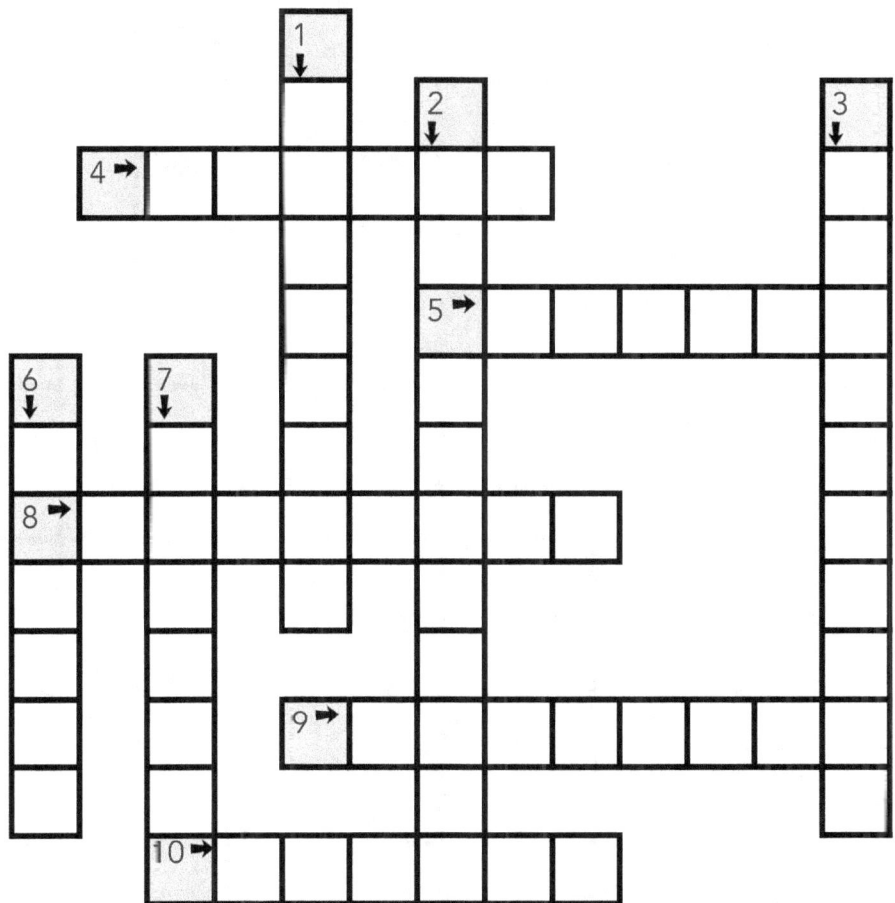

ACROSS

4. Protein aggregates associated with neurodegeneration.
5. Impaired ability to perform learned movements.
8. NMDA receptor antagonist used in treatment.
9. Excessive motor activity and emotional distress.
10. Acetylcholinesterase inhibitor medication for cognition.

DOWN

1. False fixed beliefs despite contradictory evidence
2. Dual-acting cholinesterase inhibitor drug therapy.
3. Cholinergic modulator improving neurotransmission function.
6. Glutamatergic system modulator for cognitive decline.
7. Syndrome of cognitive and functional decline.

Solution on page 103

PUZZLE 61
THE SHAKY PATH FORWARD

Clinical Cases

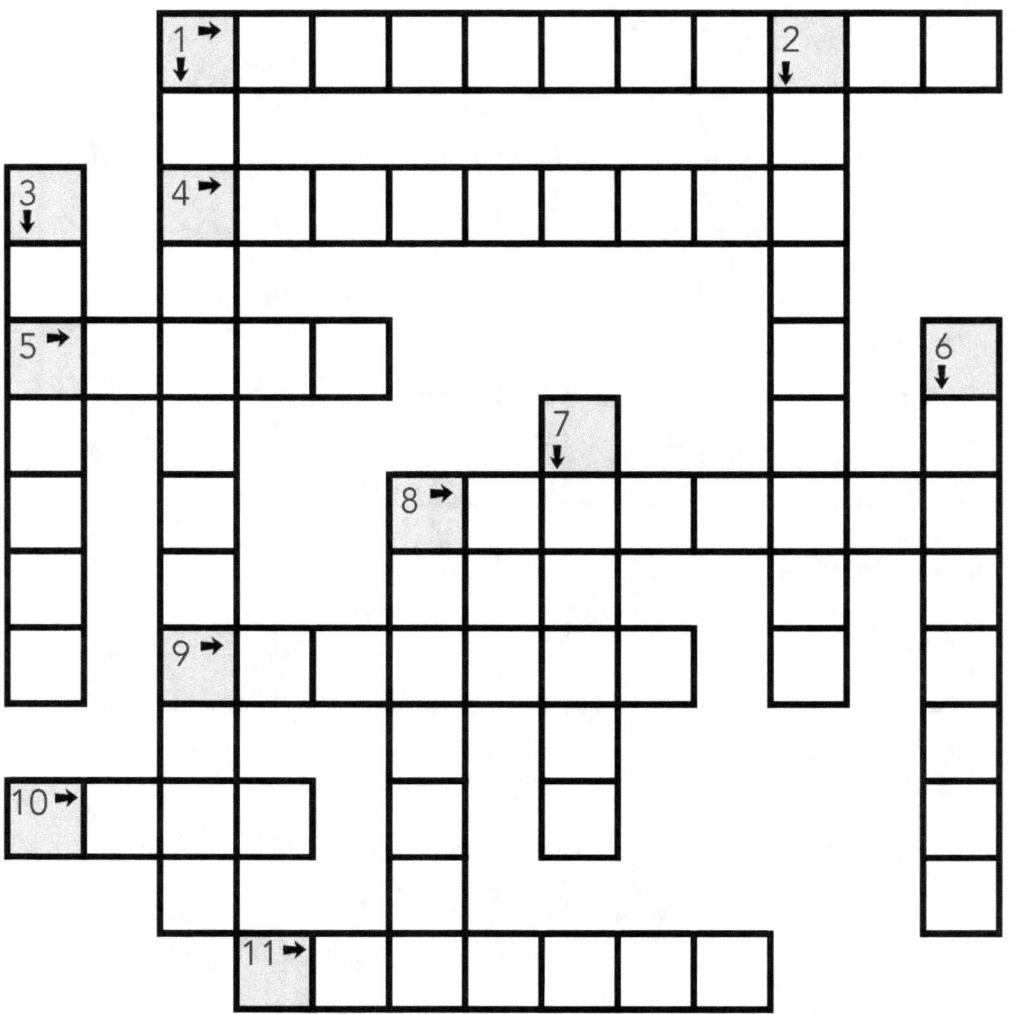

ACROSS

1. Primary area controlling voluntary movement.
4. Related to mental processes.
5. Dopamine precursor medication.
8. Sudden inability to initiate movement.
9. Body position and alignment.
10. Manner of walking or locomotion.
11. Involuntary rhythmic muscle contractions.

DOWN

1. Abnormally small handwriting.
2. Involuntary shaking or quivering.
3. Ability to maintain equilibrium.
6. Increased muscle tone and stiffness
7. Pertaining to nerves or nervous system.
8. Extreme tiredness or exhaustion.

Solution on page 103

PUZZLE 62
A BURNING QUESTION

Clinical Cases

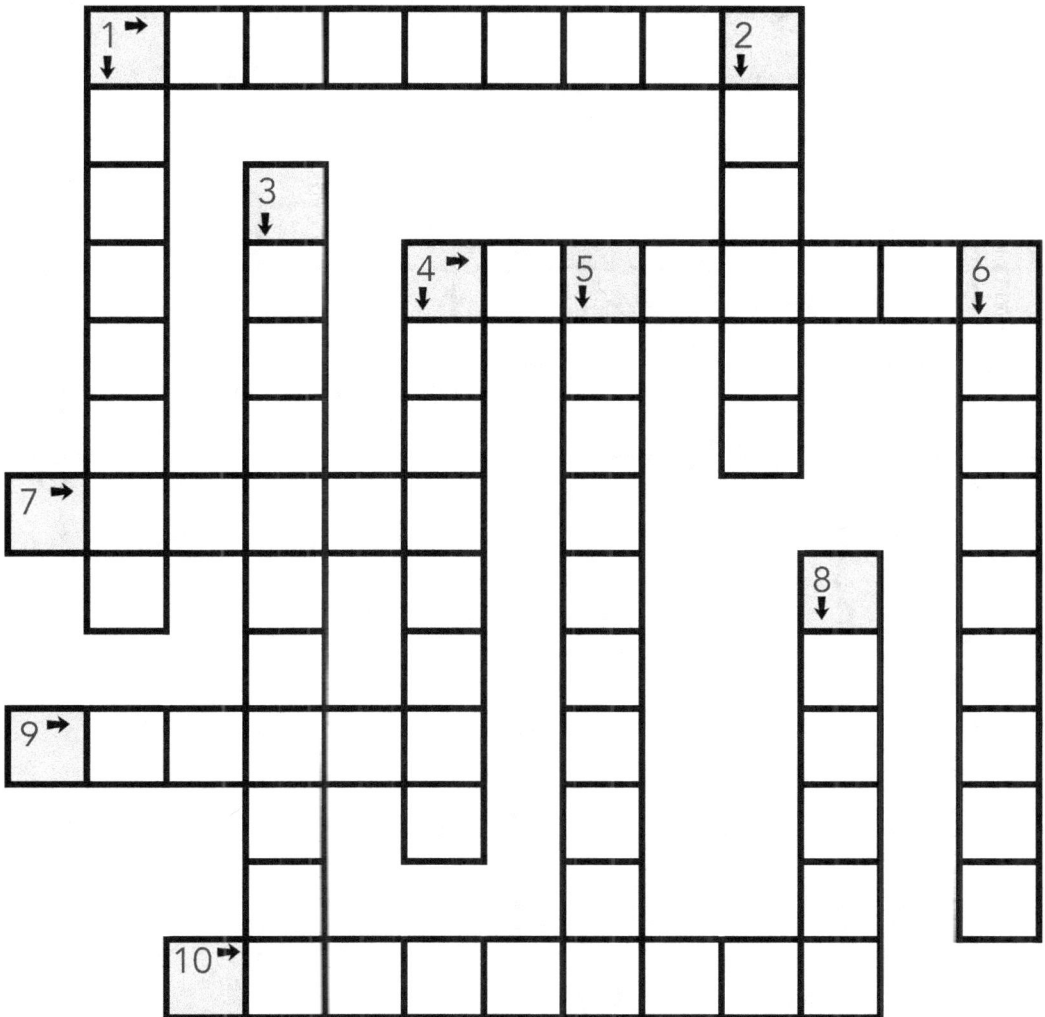

ACROSS

1. Digestive discomfort in upper abdomen.
4. Escape of blood from vessels.
7. Membrane lining gastrointestinal tract.
9. Positively charged subatomic particle.
10. Procedure to examine internal organs.

DOWN

1. First part of small intestine.
2. Having pH less than 7.
3. Hole through tissue or organ.
4. Abdominal distension causing discomfort.
5. Relating to upper central abdomen.
6. Inflammation of stomach lining.
8. Tissue sample for microscopic examination.

Solution on page 103

PUZZLE 63
THE UNSETTLED GUT

Clinical Cases

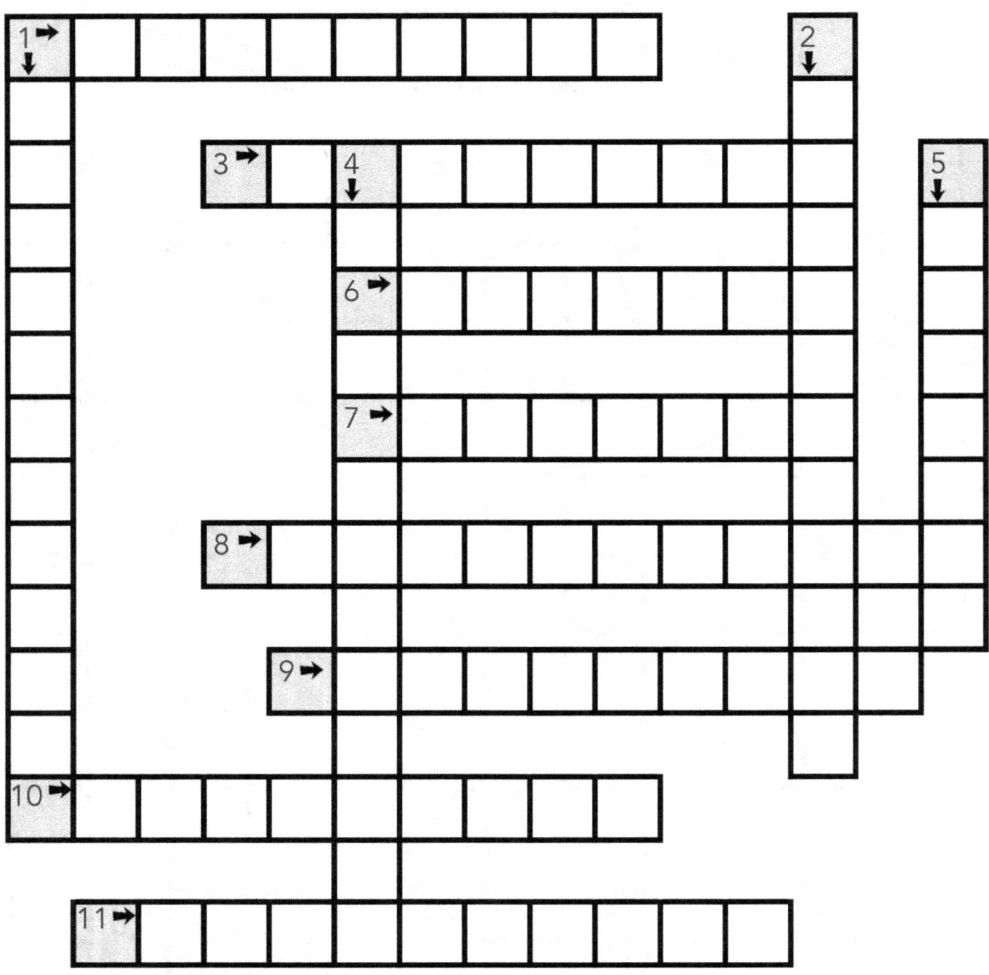

ACROSS

1. Beneficial microorganisms for digestive health.
3. Excessive intestinal gas production.
6. Frequent loose or watery stools.
7. Movement of contents through digestive tract.
8. Infrequent or difficult bowel movements.
9. Diet excluding wheat protein compound.
10. Antidiarrheal medication.
11. Endoscopic examination of large intestine.

DOWN

1. Herbal remedy for digestive discomfort.
2. Indigestible plant material aiding digestion.
4. Discomfort in stomach or intestinal region.
5. Swollen or distended feeling in abdomen.

Solution on page 104

PUZZLE 64
A LIVER'S SILENT ENEMY

Clinical Cases

ACROSS

1. Bile flow obstruction within liver.
2. Enzyme indicating liver cell damage.
5. Advanced scarring of liver tissue.
7. Yellowish pigment in bile metabolism.
8. Viral presence in bloodstream.
9. Immune protein with antiviral properties.
10. Abnormal enlargement of the spleen.

DOWN

1. Cell-signaling proteins in immune response.
3. Fluid accumulation in peritoneal cavity.
4. Yellowing of skin and eyes.
6. Antiviral medication for RNA viruses.

Solution on page 104

PUZZLE 65
THE IMMUNE SYSTEM'S HIDDEN BATTLE

Clinical Cases

ACROSS

1. Protein that binds specific molecules.
4. Process of viral genome duplication.
8. Describing infections in immunocompromised patients.
9. Antiretroviral medication class abbreviation.
10. Patient's commitment to treatment regimen.

DOWN

2. Cell signaling protein in immune responses.
3. Enzyme that breaks down proteins.
4. RNA virus that reverse transcribes DNA.
5. Develop detectable antibodies after infection.
6. Rare cancer affecting blood vessels.
7. Antiviral drug pharmacokinetic enhancer.

Solution on page 104

PUZZLE 66
A PERSISTENT SHADOW IN THE LUNGS

Clinical Cases

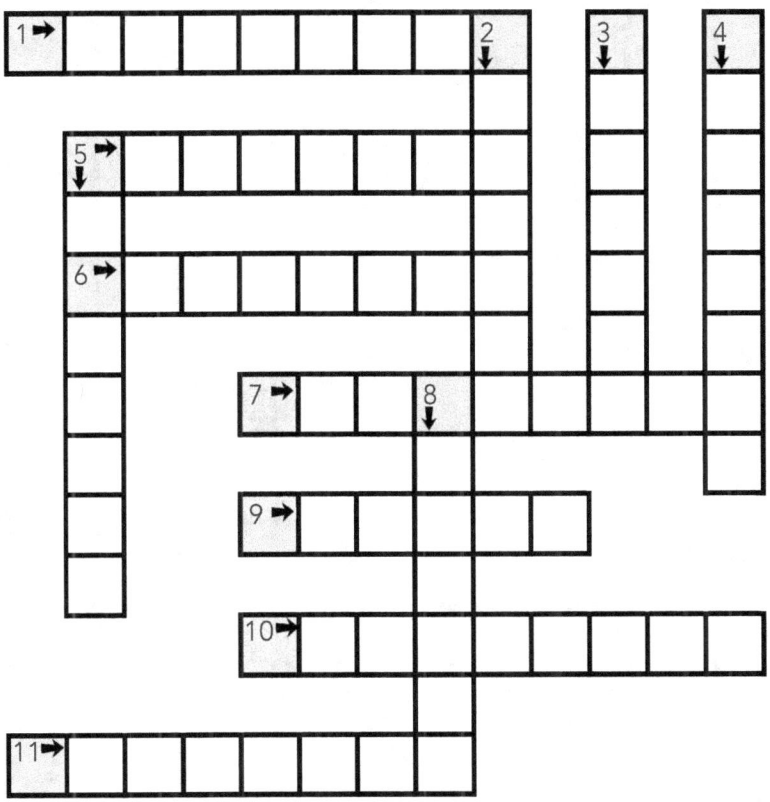

ACROSS

1. First-line antibiotic for mycobacterial infections.
5. Airborne particles carrying infectious agents.
6. Antibiotic targeting bacterial RNA polymerase.
7. Preventive measure for contagious patients.
9. Expectorated respiratory tract secretions.
10. Organized collection of immune cells.
11. Describing lung lesions with hollowed spaces.

DOWN

2. Subjective sensation of breathing difficulty.
3. Rod-shaped bacteria visible under microscope.
4. Reflexive expulsion of airway irritants.
5. Metabolically inactive state of microorganisms.
8. Asymptomatic period following initial infection.

Solution on page 104

PUZZLE 67
THE THIN RED LINE

Clinical Cases

ACROSS

1. Bone marrow failure condition.
6. Difficulty breathing symptom.
7. Large, immature red blood cell type.
8. Intravenous blood product administration.
10. Abnormal paleness of skin.
11. Metal ion binding therapy.

DOWN

2. Essential vitamin for erythropoiesis.
3. Iron storage protein measurement.
4. Small red blood cell characteristic.
5. Red blood cell volume percentage.
9. B vitamin crucial for DNA synthesis.

Solution on page 104

PUZZLE 68
A GLAND'S WILD RIDE

Clinical Cases

ACROSS

1. Anatomical region anterior to tibia bone.
7. Synthetic hormone replacement medication.
8. Radioisotope used in nuclear medicine imaging.
9. Medication inhibiting hormone production.

DOWN

1. Sensation of rapid or irregular heartbeats.
2. Abnormally slow heart rate condition.
3. Inflammation of endocrine gland in neck.
4. Severe form of hypothyroidism complication.
5. Abnormally rapid heart rate condition.
6. Normal glandular function state.

Solution on page 104

PUZZLE 69
A MIND IN TURMOIL

Clinical Cases

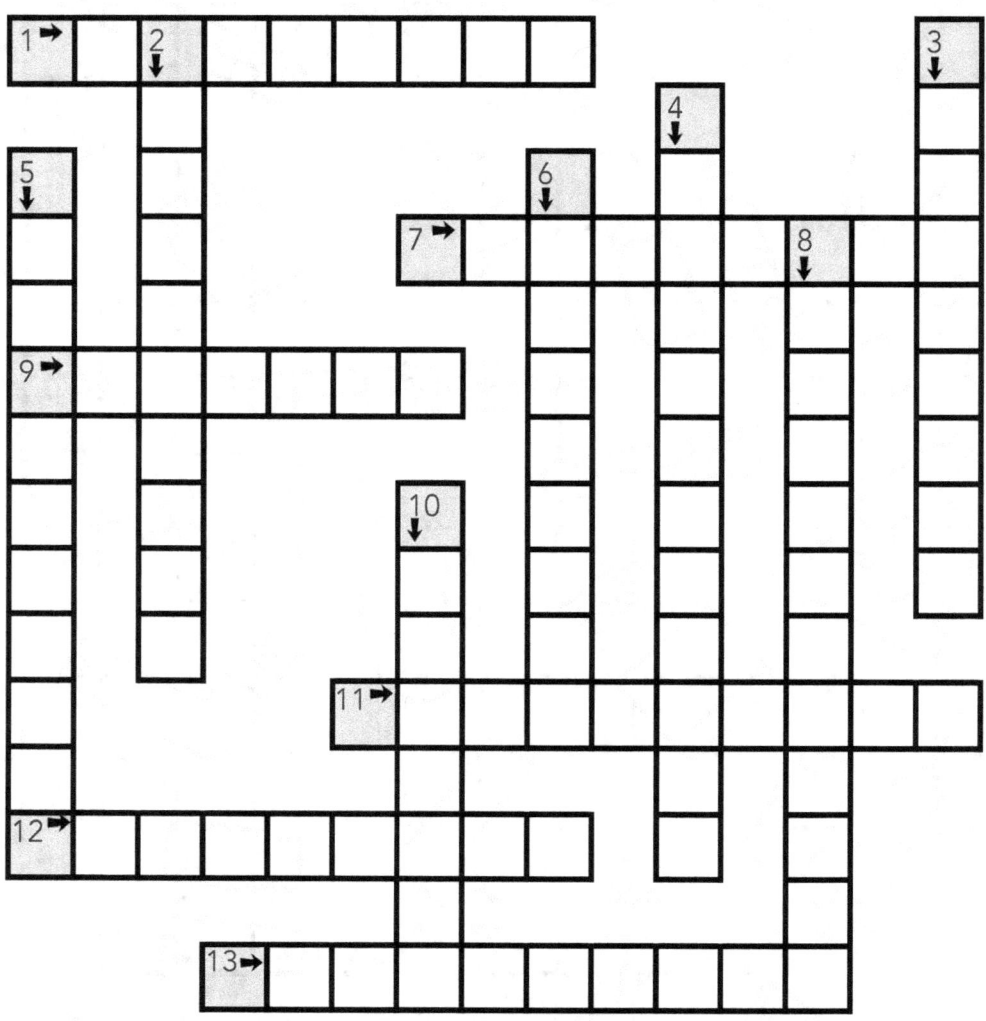

ACROSS

1. Persistent mild depressive disorder.
7. Recurring, intrusive thoughts or behaviors.
9. Profound sense of hopelessness.
11. Therapeutic dialogue for mental health.
12. Neurotransmitter affecting mood regulation.
13. Persistent feeling of sadness.

DOWN

2. Personal sense of worth.
3. Inability to feel pleasure.
4. Persistent urge for movement.
5. Present-moment awareness practice.
6. Withdrawal from social interactions.
8. Heightened sensitivity to stimuli.
10. Chronic difficulty falling asleep.

Solution on page 104

PUZZLE 70
A RASH DECISION

Clinical Cases

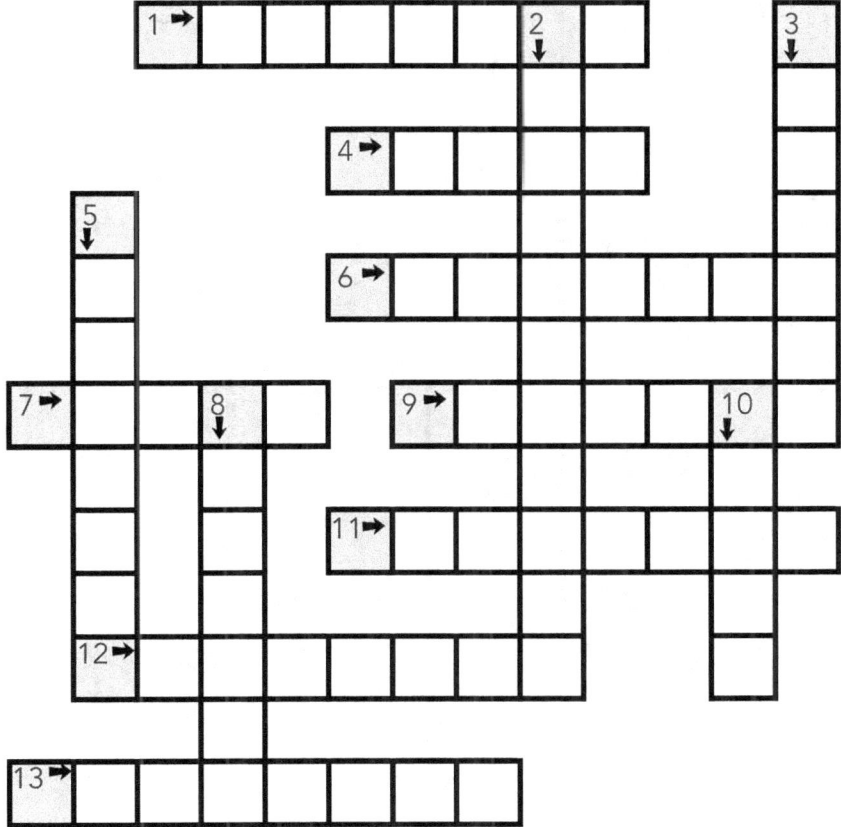

ACROSS

1. Pus-filled lesions often seen in bacterial skin infections.
4. Circumscribed area of altered skin color or texture.
6. Medical term for severe itching sensation on skin.
7. Genetic tendency to develop allergic diseases like asthma.
9. Raised, flat-topped lesions larger than papules on skin.
11. Small fluid-filled blisters occurring on skin surface.
12. Substance triggering exaggerated immune response in body.
13. Formation of hardened layer over healing skin wound.

DOWN

2. Self-inflicted scratching damage to skin's outer layers.
3. Abnormally dry skin condition causing roughness and scaling.
5. Redness of skin due to capillary dilation.
8. Small, solid, raised lesions on skin under 1cm.
10. Swelling caused by excess fluid in body tissues.

Solution on page 105

PUZZLE 71
A VEIN'S TREACHEROUS PATH

Clinical Cases

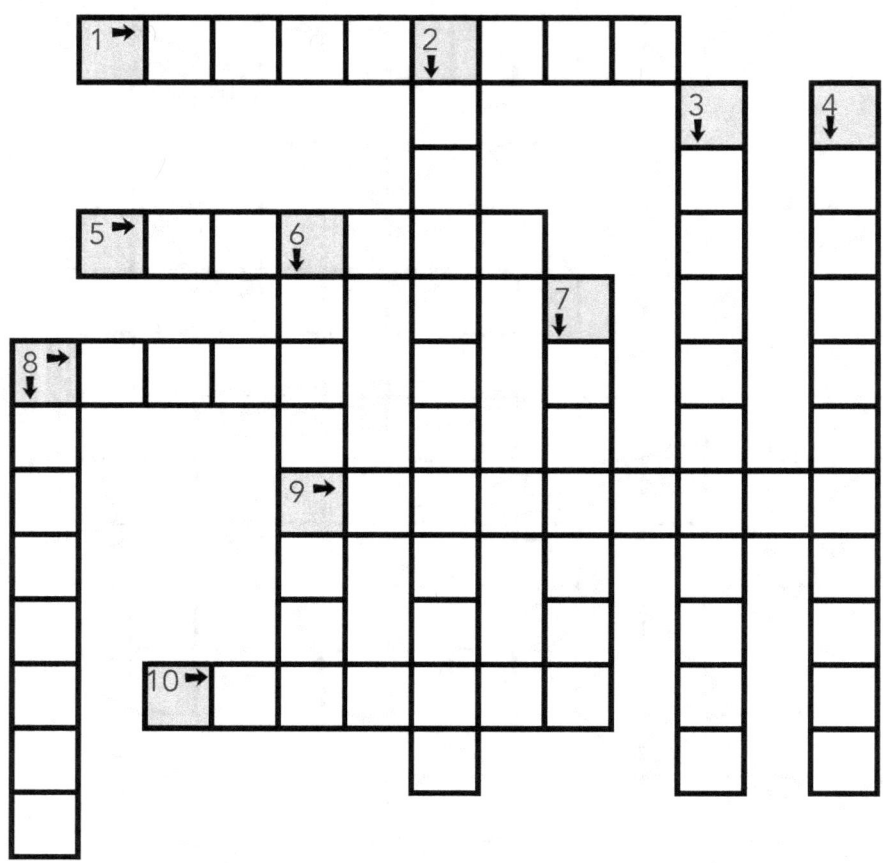

ACROSS

1. Abnormally rapid breathing rate, often exceeding 20 breaths per minute.
5. Sudden, brief loss of consciousness due to reduced blood flow.
8. Abnormal accumulation of fluid in body tissues or cavities.
9. Difficulty breathing when lying flat, relieved by sitting up.
10. Subjective sensation of breathing difficulty or shortness of breath.

DOWN

2. Awareness of forceful, rapid, or irregular heartbeats.
3. Abnormally low blood pressure, potentially causing dizziness or fainting.
4. Abnormally rapid heart rate, typically exceeding 100 beats per minute.
6. Bluish discoloration of skin due to poor blood oxygenation.
7. Inadequate oxygen supply at the tissue level.
8. Redness of skin caused by increased blood flow.

Solution on page 105

PUZZLE 72
THE SILENT BLOOD THIEF

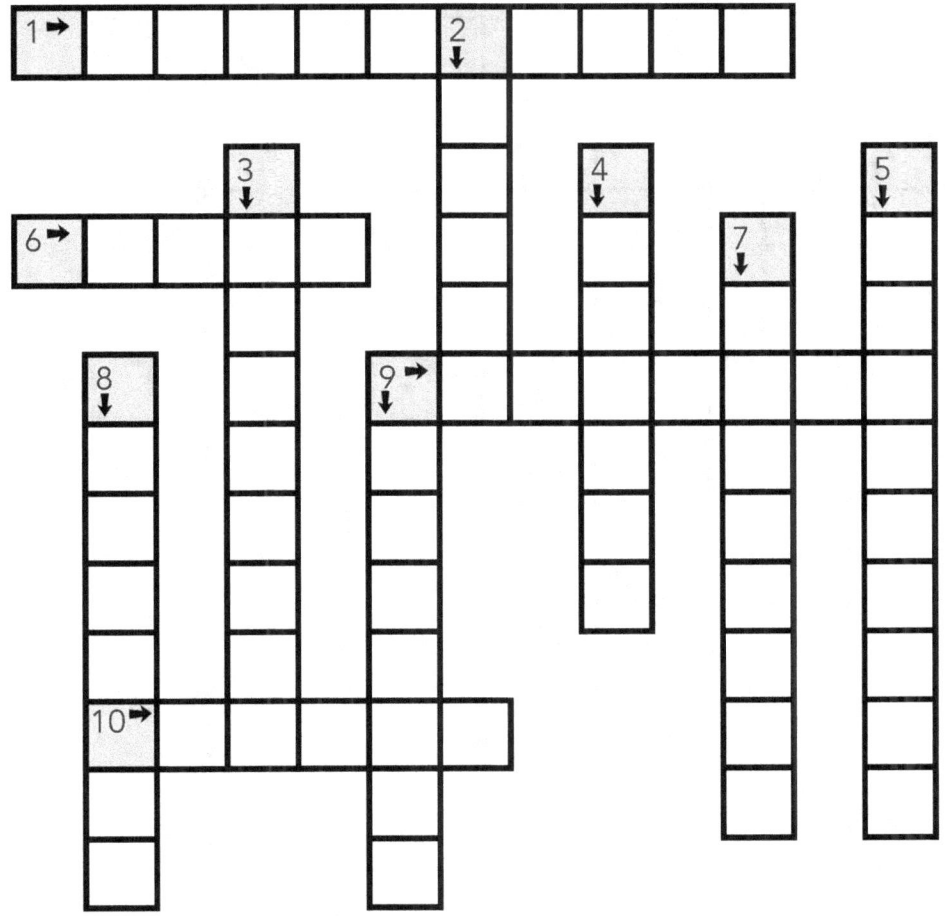

ACROSS

1. Abnormally low count of specific white blood cells.
6. Elevated body temperature associated with immune response.
9. Discoloration of skin due to blood vessel damage.
10. Condition of insufficient healthy red blood cells.

DOWN

2. Unhealthy pale appearance of skin or mucous membranes.
3. Tiny round spots on skin caused by bleeding.
4. Persistent tiredness and lack of energy in patients.
5. Unintentional decrease in body mass over time.
7. Medical term for bleeding from the nasal passages.
8. Discomfort in skeletal structure, often deep-seated ache.
9. Escape of blood from damaged blood vessels internally.

Solution on page 105

PUZZLE 73
A CLOUDED MIND

Clinical Cases

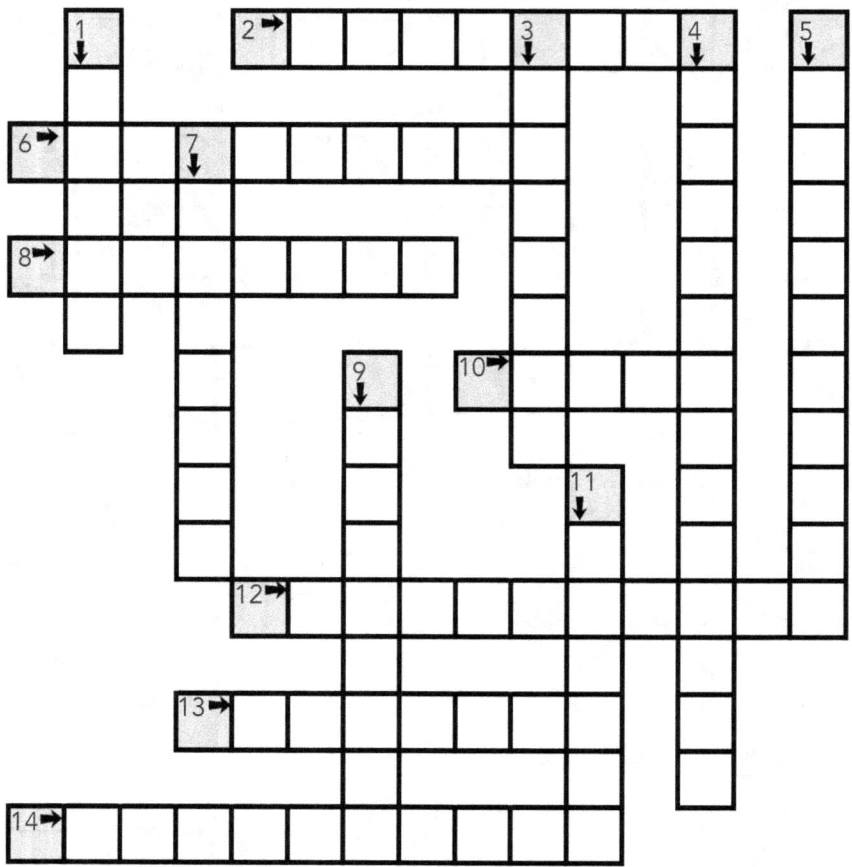

ACROSS

2. Altered mental state affecting cognition and awareness.
6. Neck flexion test assessing spinal cord irritation.
8. Visual disturbance characterized by perceiving double images.
10. Elevated body temperature indicating systemic inflammatory response.
12. Abnormally rapid heart rate exceeding 100 beats.
13. Forceful expulsion of stomach contents through mouth.
14. Optic disc swelling due to increased intracranial.

DOWN

1. Leg extension test evaluating spinal nerve root.
3. Sudden, uncontrolled electrical disturbances in the brain.
4. Stiff neck associated with cervical muscle.
5. Increased sensitivity to light causing ocular discomfort.
7. Acute confusional state characterized by disorientation and cognitive impairment.
9. Small, round, purple spots caused by capillary bleeding.
11. Muscle pain or tenderness often associated with.

Solution on page 105

PUZZLE 74
THE HIDDEN UTERINE BATTLE

Clinical Cases

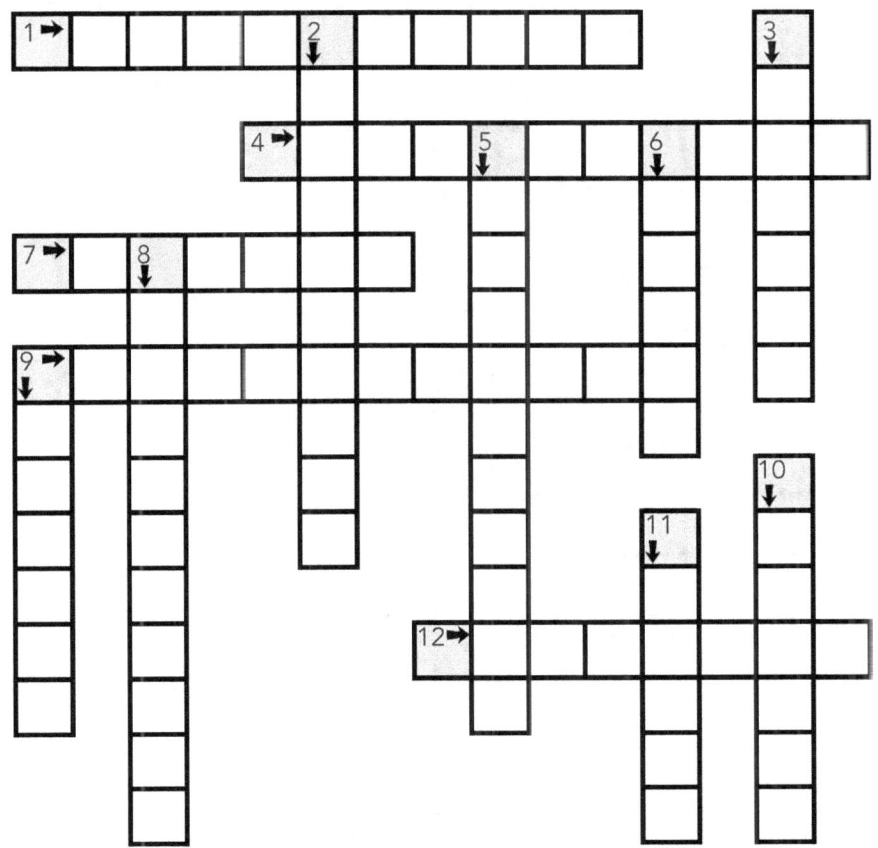

ACROSS

1. Inability to conceive after one year of unprotected intercourse.
4. Relating to the inner lining of the uterus.
7. Small, solid masses of tissue in organs or glands.
9. Painful menstruation affecting reproductive and urinary systems.
12. Formation of excess fibrous connective tissue in organs.

DOWN

2. Sensitivity to touch in specific areas of the body
3. Pertaining to female reproductive organs producing ova and hormones.
5. Abnormally heavy or prolonged menstrual bleeding in women.
6. Related to the terminal part of the digestive tract.
8. Pain experienced during sexual intercourse in pelvic region.
9. Painful or difficult urination often indicating urinary tract issues.
10. Persistent tiredness and lack of energy affecting daily activities.
11. Removal and examination of tissue for diagnostic purposes.

Solution on page 105

PUZZLE 75
AN OVERFLOW OF RED

Clinical Cases

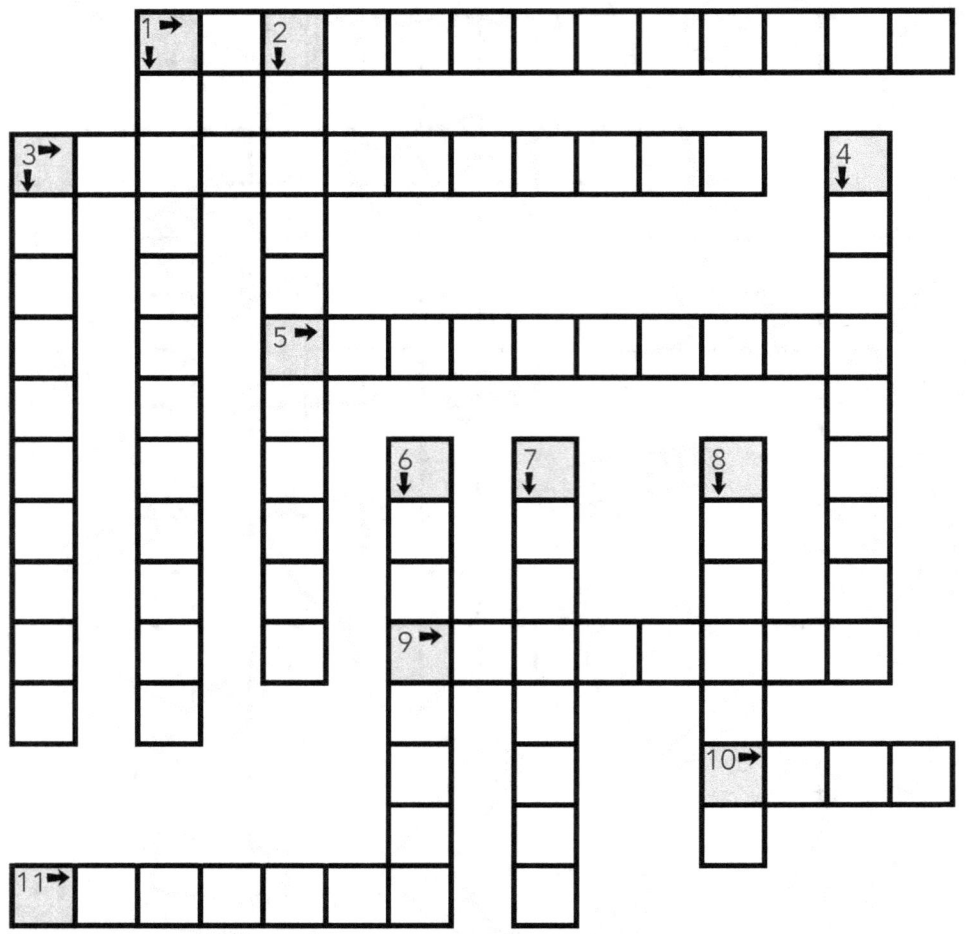

ACROSS

1. Elevated serum uric acid levels in blood.
3. Persistently high arterial blood pressure condition.
5. Formation of blood clots within blood vessels.
9. Perception of ringing or buzzing sounds in ears.
10. Inflammatory arthritis caused by uric acid crystals.
11. Subjective feeling of breathing difficulty or shortness.

DOWN

1. Abnormal enlargement of the liver organ.
2. Abnormal sensation of tingling, numbness, or burning.
3. Excessive bleeding from damaged blood vessels.
4. Medical term for nosebleed or nasal hemorrhage.
6. Excess of blood or fluid in body tissues.
7. Bluish discoloration of skin due to deoxygenation.
8. Sensation of spinning or loss of balance.

Solution on page 105

PUZZLE 76
THE DAWN OF ANTIBIOTICS

Medical innovations and breakthroughs

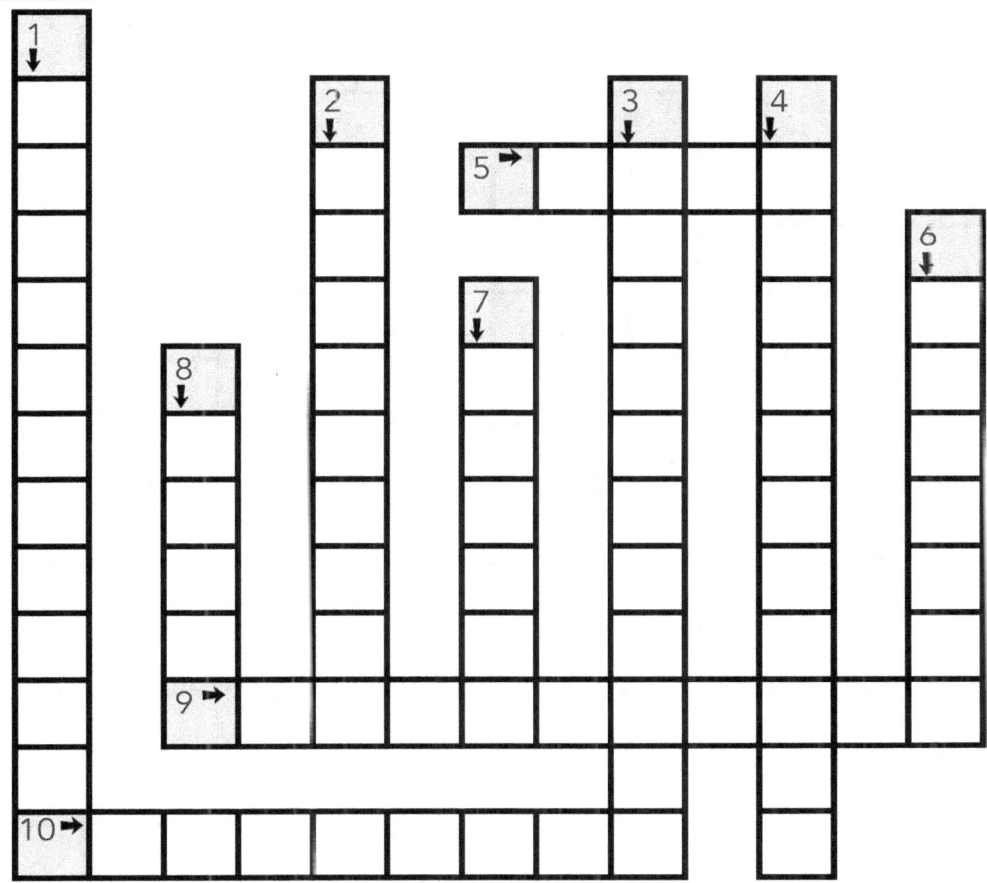

ACROSS

5. A type of virus that infects and kills bacteria, now being explored as an alternative to traditional antibiotics.
9. The process of reversing bacterial resistance, allowing antibiotics to regain effectiveness against resistant strains.
10. Bacteria resistant to multiple antibiotics.

DOWN

1. Tiny particles engineered to deliver antibiotics directly to infected areas, increasing the drug's effectiveness.
2. Last-resort antibiotics for resistant bacterial infections.
3. Proteins produced by bacteria that kill or inhibit the growth of other bacteria, showing potential as a new class of antibiotics.
4. Study of microbial genes for new antibiotic discovery.
6. Target of many antibiotics, halts bacterial protein synthesis.
7. A breakthrough antibiotic discovered using AI, capable of killing antibiotic-resistant bacteria, including E. coli.
8. Gene-editing tool used to fight antibiotic resistance.

Solution on page 105

PUZZLE 77
CRACKING THE CODE

Medical innovations and breakthroughs

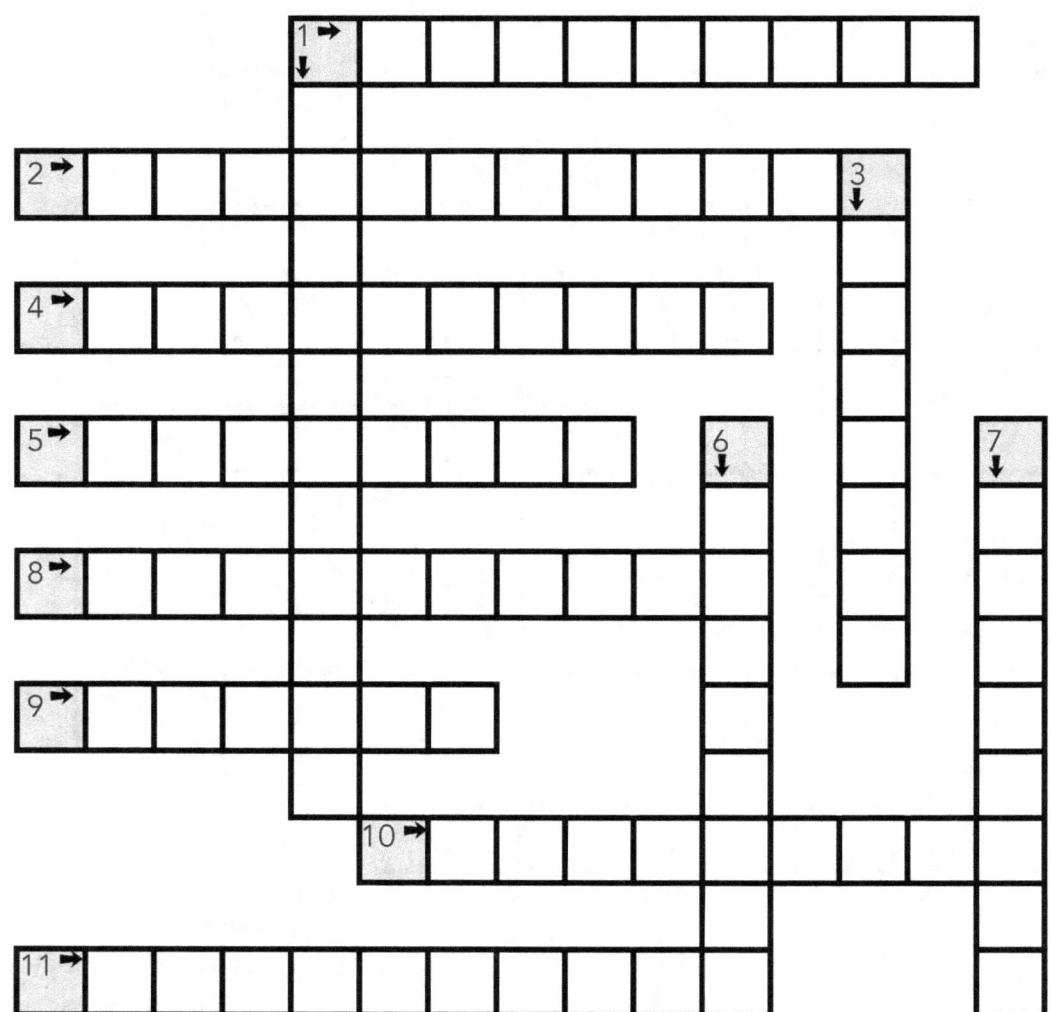

ACROSS
1. DNA analysis technique.
2. Chromosome location identification method.
4. Genetic material transfer treatment.
5. Undifferentiated cellular building blocks.
8. DNA and RNA structural units.
9. Alternative gene forms.
10. Genetically transmitted trait characteristic.
11. Gene expression regulation study.

DOWN
1. Non-reproductive body cells.
3. Organism's genetic constitution.
6. Complementary nucleotide duos.
7. Observable genetic trait manifestation.

Solution on page 106

PUZZLE 78
SUPPLEMENTS UNCOVERED

Medical innovations and breakthroughs

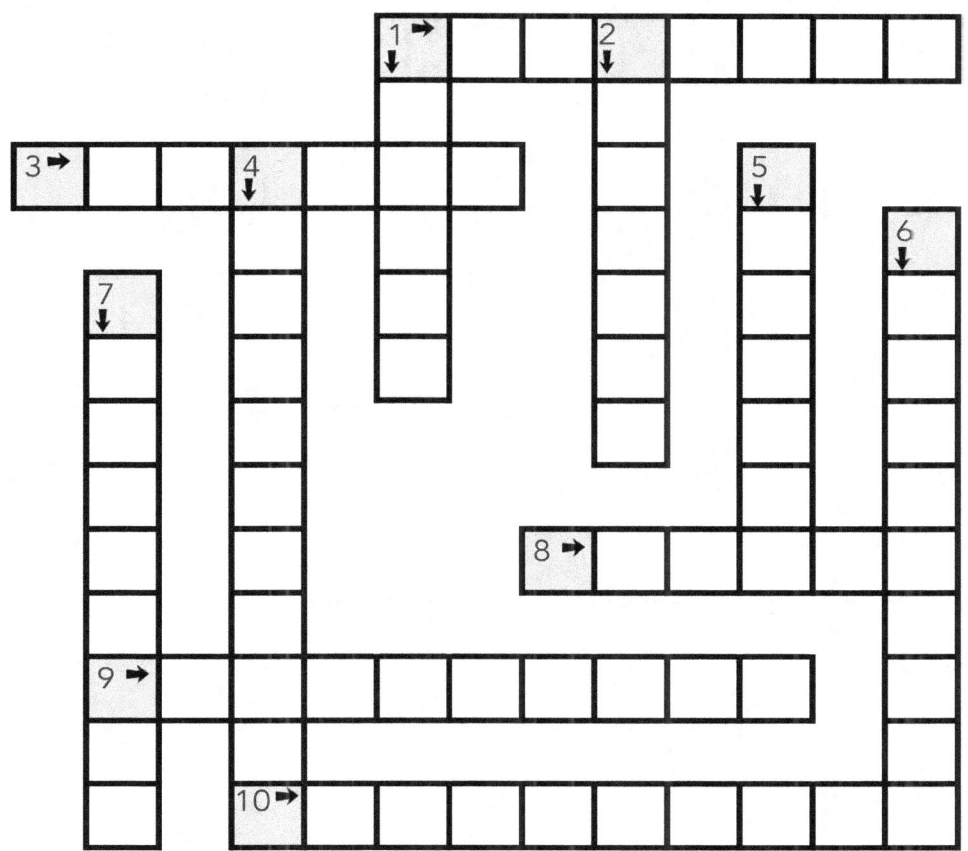

ACROSS

1. Herb used to combat fatigue and enhance cognitive function.
3. Proprietary yeast beta-glucan supplement for immune system support.
8. Dietary supplement designation indicating absence of genetic modification.
9. Berry extract commonly used to boost immune system.
10. Class of herbs that help body adapt to stress.

DOWN

1. Medicinal mushroom traditionally used to support immune function.
2. Proprietary sleep supplement blend containing melatonin and herbs.
4. Ayurvedic herb known for stress reduction properties.
5. Root used to improve energy and cognitive performance.
6. Cognitive-enhancing substances that may improve mental function.
7. Fungus used in supplements to boost energy levels.

Solution on page 106

PUZZLE 78
THE BIRTH OF MODERN SURGERY

Medical innovations and breakthroughs

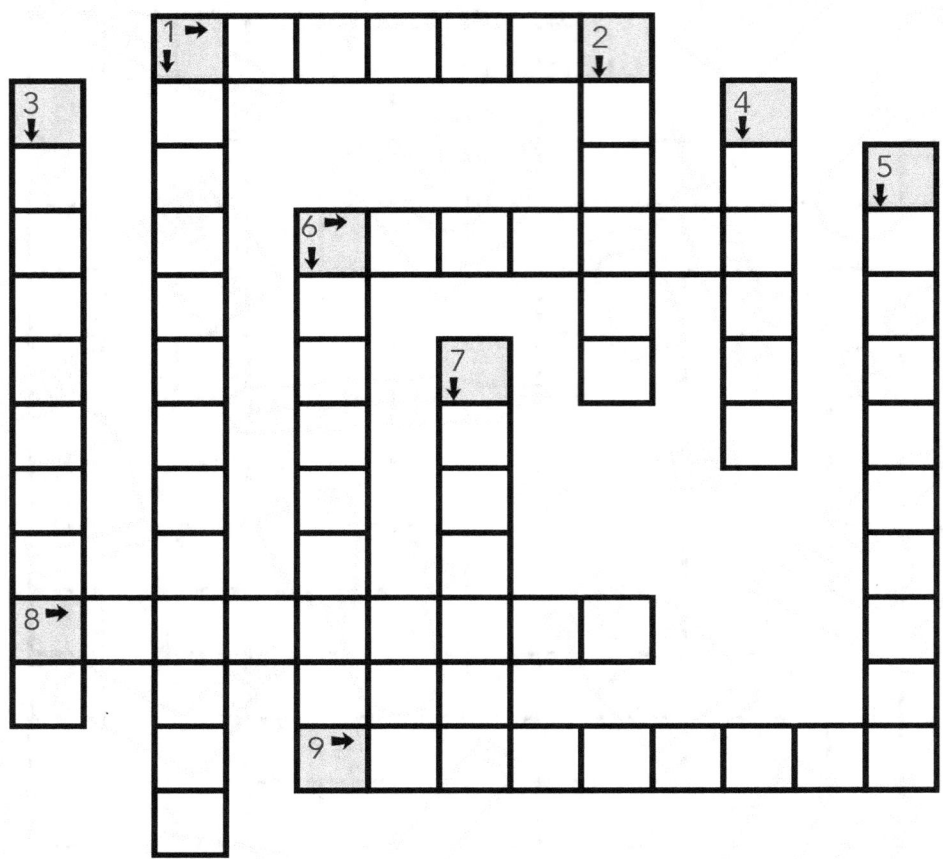

ACROSS

1. Surgical cutting instrument with a sharp blade.
6. Free from pathogenic microorganisms.
8. Instrument used to hold back tissues during surgery.
9. Procedure to examine internal organs using a camera.

DOWN

1. Process of eliminating all microorganisms from instruments.
2. Surgeon who pioneered antiseptic surgical techniques.
3. Early anesthetic agent used in surgical procedures.
4. Swiss surgeon known for thyroid surgery innovations.
5. Surgical incision into the abdominal cavity.
6. Device using high-pressure steam for sterilization.
7. American surgeon who developed radical mastectomy technique.

Solution on page 106

84

PUZZLE 79
PIONEERING THE PACEMAKER

Medical innovations and breakthroughs

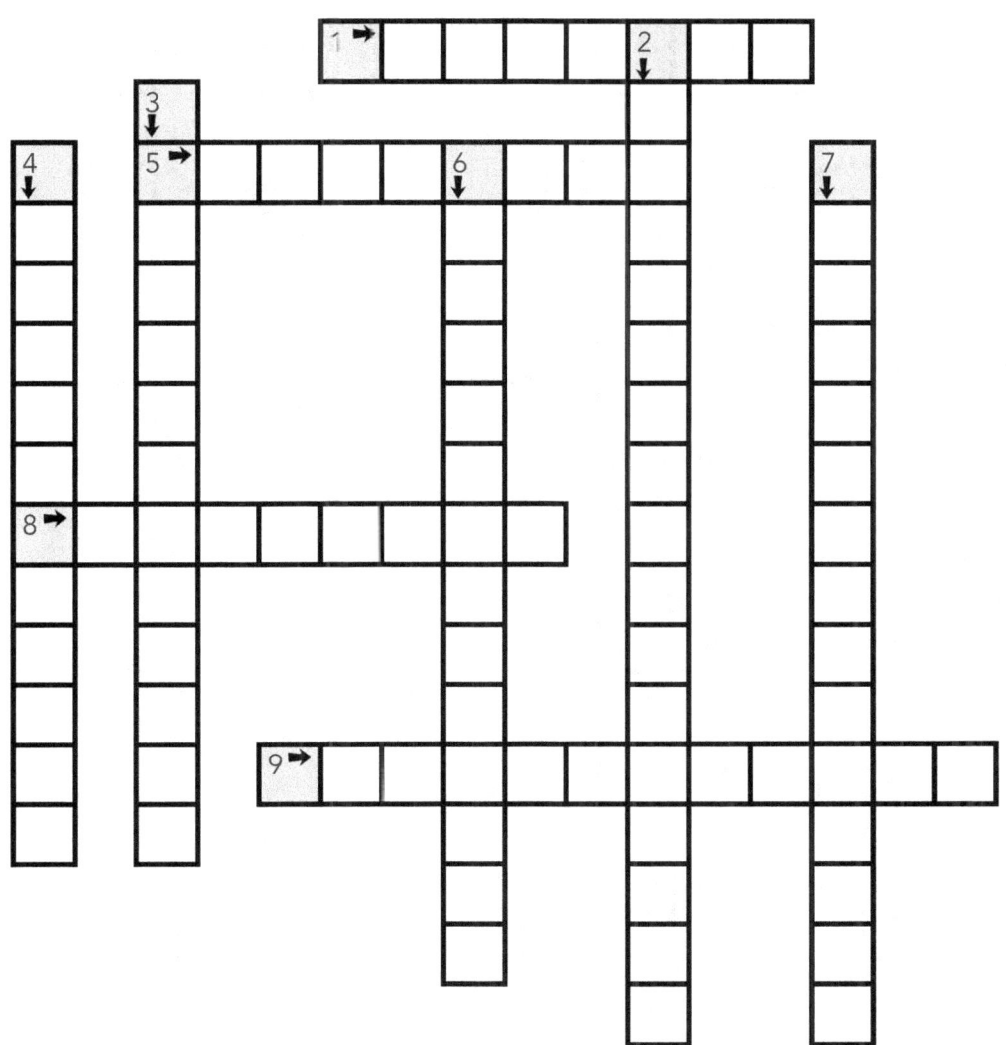

ACROSS

1. Miniature pacemaker design without traditional transvenous leads.
5. Conductive component for sensing cardiac electrical activity.
8. Wireless data transmission system in cardiac devices.
9. Light-energy conversion principle for powering implantable devices.

DOWN

2. Study of heart's electrical properties and conduction.
3. Device delivering electric shock to restore normal rhythm.
4. Surgical procedure for inserting cardiac devices subcutaneously.
6. Restoration of cardiac cell membrane potential post-contraction.
7. Coordinated timing of pacemaker pulses with cardiac cycle.

Solution on page 106

PUZZLE 80
A NEW LOOK INSIDE

Medical innovations and breakthroughs

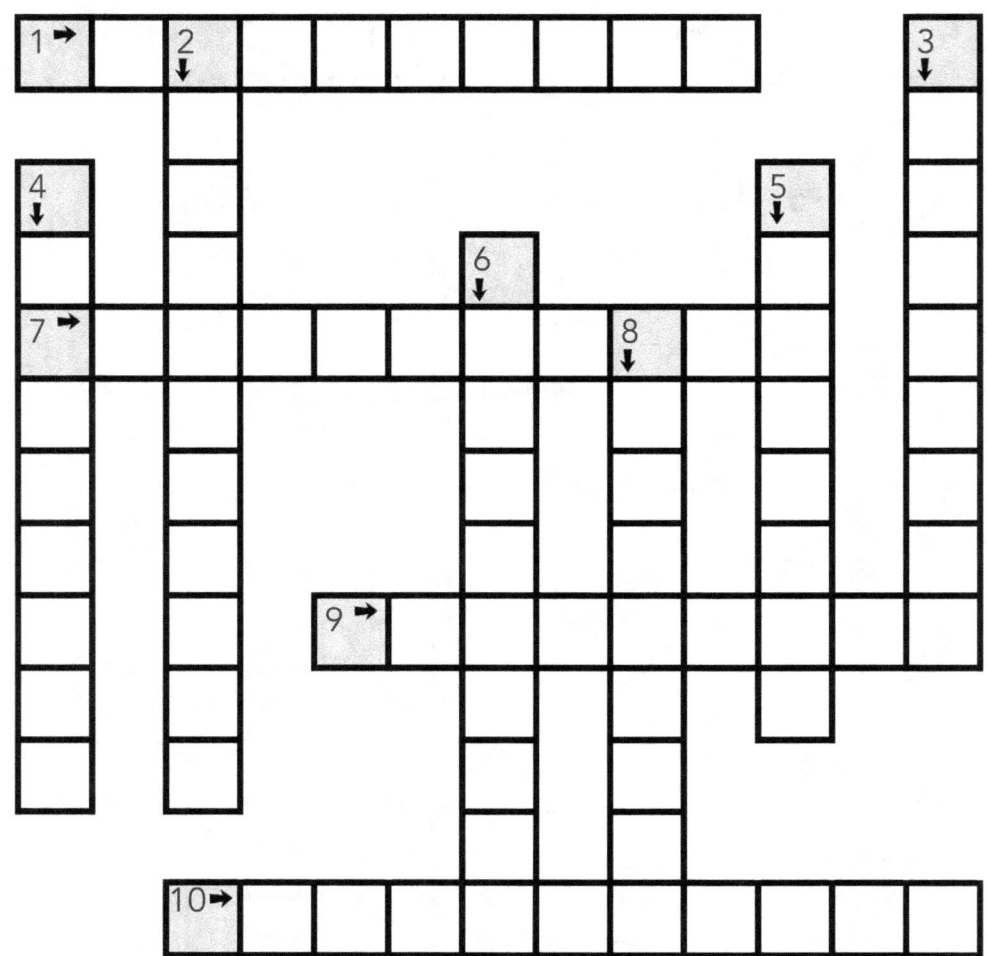

ACROSS

1. Deviation of X-rays from straight path in tissue.
7. Particle accelerator producing high-energy X-rays for imaging.
9. Specialized X-ray exam for early breast cancer detection.
10. Real-time X-ray imaging technique for dynamic body processes.

DOWN

2. Reduction of X-ray beam intensity through matter.
3. X-ray procedure to visualize blood vessels using contrast.
4. Measurement and calculation of radiation dose in tissue.
5. Partially shaded area at edge of X-ray beam.
6. Device that narrows X-ray beam for focused imaging.
8. Extraction of quantitative features from medical images.

PUZZLE 81
VACCINES THAT CHANGED THE WORLD

Medical innovations and breakthroughs

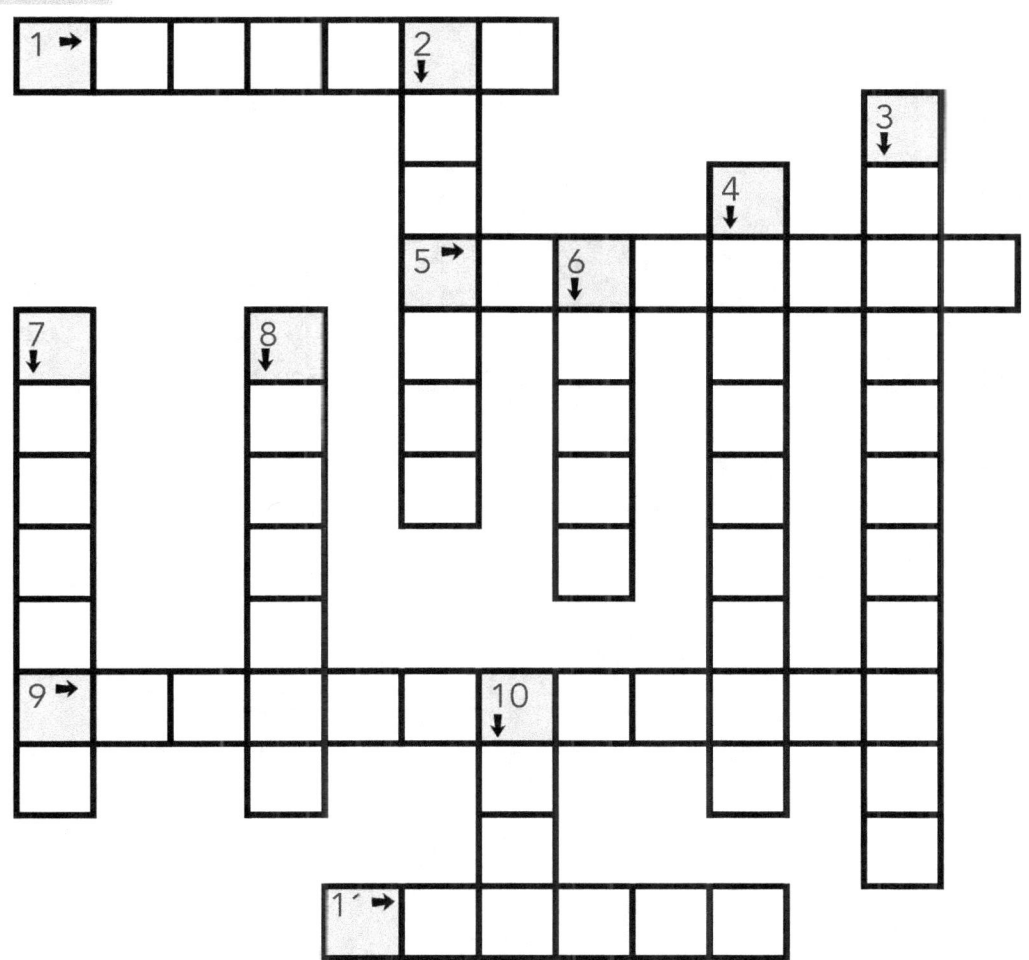

ACROSS

1. Meningococcal B vaccine developed to prevent serogroup B infection.
5. Global disease outbreak affecting multiple countries or continents.
9. Process of inducing immunity through vaccine administration.
11. Ebola vaccine approved for use in outbreaks.

DOWN

2. Respiratory syncytial virus prefusion F protein-based vaccine.
3. Mosquito-borne viral disease targeted by experimental vaccines.
4. First licensed vaccine against dengue fever.
6. Lung cancer subtype targeted by immunotherapy vaccines.
7. Hepatitis E vaccine developed and licensed in China.
8. Vaccine-preventable disease caused by Clostridium tetani toxin.
10. Zika purified inactivated virus vaccine candidate.

Solution on page 106

PUZZLE 82
REVIVING HEALTH WITH AI

Medical innovations and breakthroughs

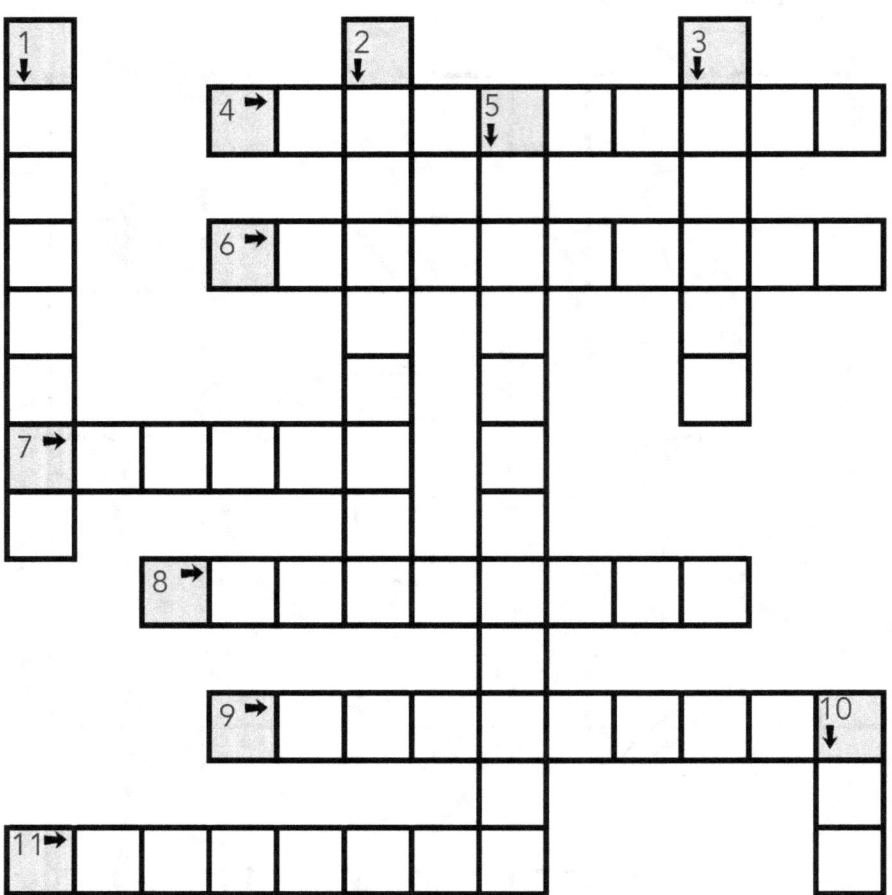

ACROSS

4. Statistical technique to assess AI model performance.
6. Data preparation step for machine learning algorithms.
7. Group studied in longitudinal clinical research design.
8. Measurable indicator of disease state or condition.
9. Capability of AI to forecast medical outcomes.
11. Mathematical representation of biological systems for analysis.

DOWN

1. Measure of correctness in AI diagnostic predictions.
2. Step-by-step procedure for solving diagnostic problems.
3. Extracting valuable patterns from large medical datasets.
5. Neural network approach for complex diagnostic tasks.
10. Digital system for storing and managing patient records.

Solution on page 106

PUZZLE 83
REGENERATIVE REVOLUTION

Medical innovations and breakthroughs

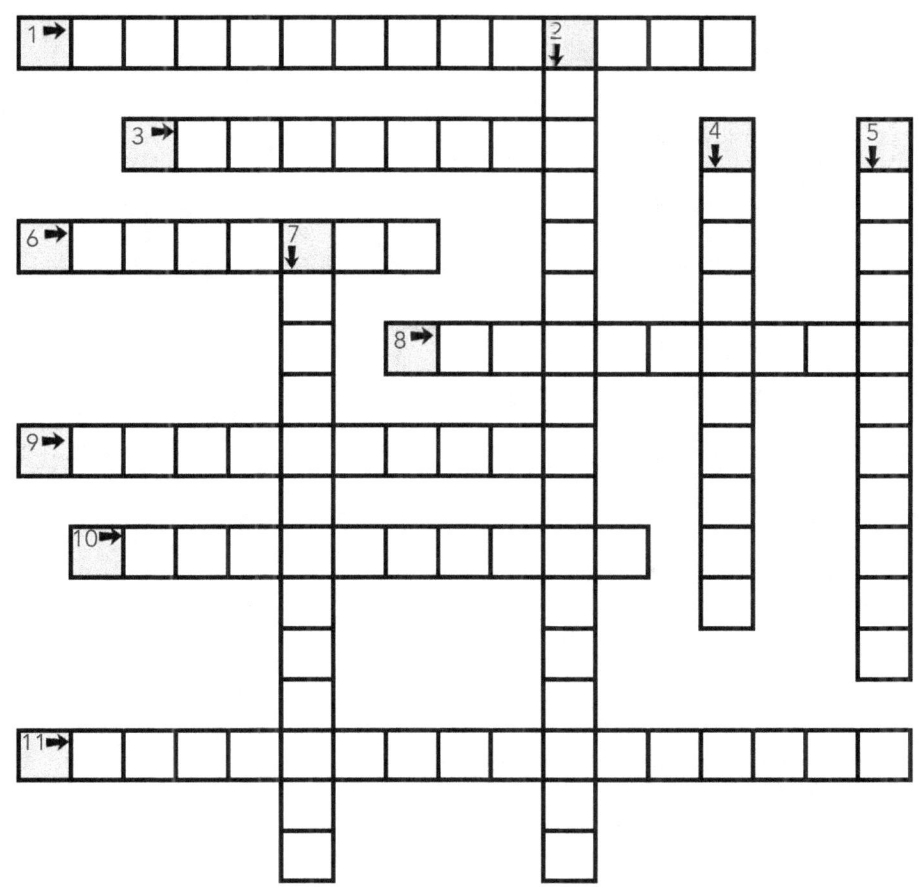

ACROSS

1. Surgical approach to restore form and function post-injury.
3. Undifferentiated cells capable of developing into specialized types.
6. Containing genetic material from two or more organisms.
8. Bone-forming cell responsible for synthesizing new osseous tissue.
9. Biocompatible structure supporting three-dimensional tissue growth.
10. Technique for fabricating tissue constructs using 3D printing.
11. Process of adding specific biomolecules to enhance material properties.

DOWN

2. Interdisciplinary field combining cells, scaffolds, and bioactive factors.
4. Derived from and transferred back to same individual.
5. Treatment approach using living cells to repair tissues.
7. Process of reverting differentiated cells to pluripotent state.

Solution on page 106

PUZZLE 84
INNOVATION IN SURGICAL INTERVENTIONS

Medical innovations and breakthroughs

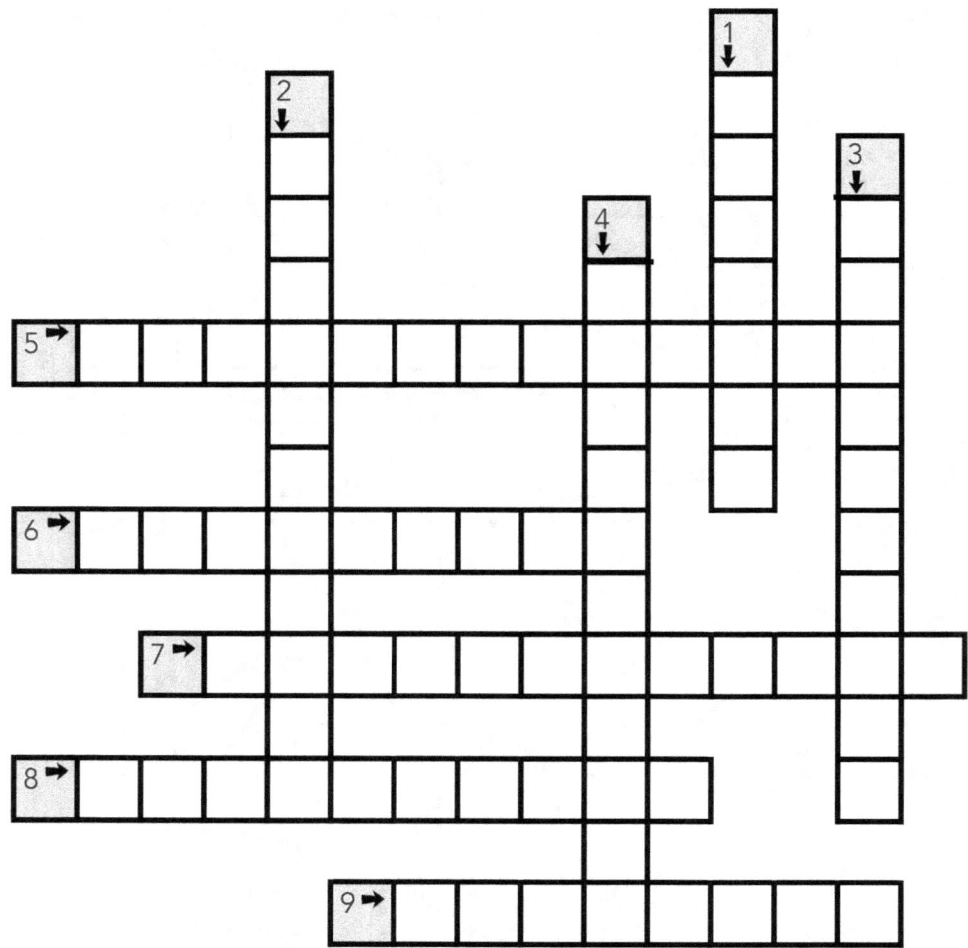

ACROSS

5. Surgical monitoring technique using real-time imaging during procedures.
6. Innovative closure method eliminating traditional wound stitching techniques.
7. Minimally invasive approach for cardiac valve replacement procedures.
8. Tissue destruction technique utilizing extreme cold for tumor.
9. Minimally invasive diagnostic and therapeutic procedure using optical.

DOWN

1. Computer-assisted surgical systems enhancing precision and dexterity.
2. Engineered substances designed for medical implants and devices.
3. Remote surgical procedures performed using advanced telecommunication technologies.
4. Specialized wound closure materials with embedded sensing capabilities.

Solution on page 107

PUZZLE 85
REVOLUTIONIZING CANCER CARE

Medical innovations and breakthroughs

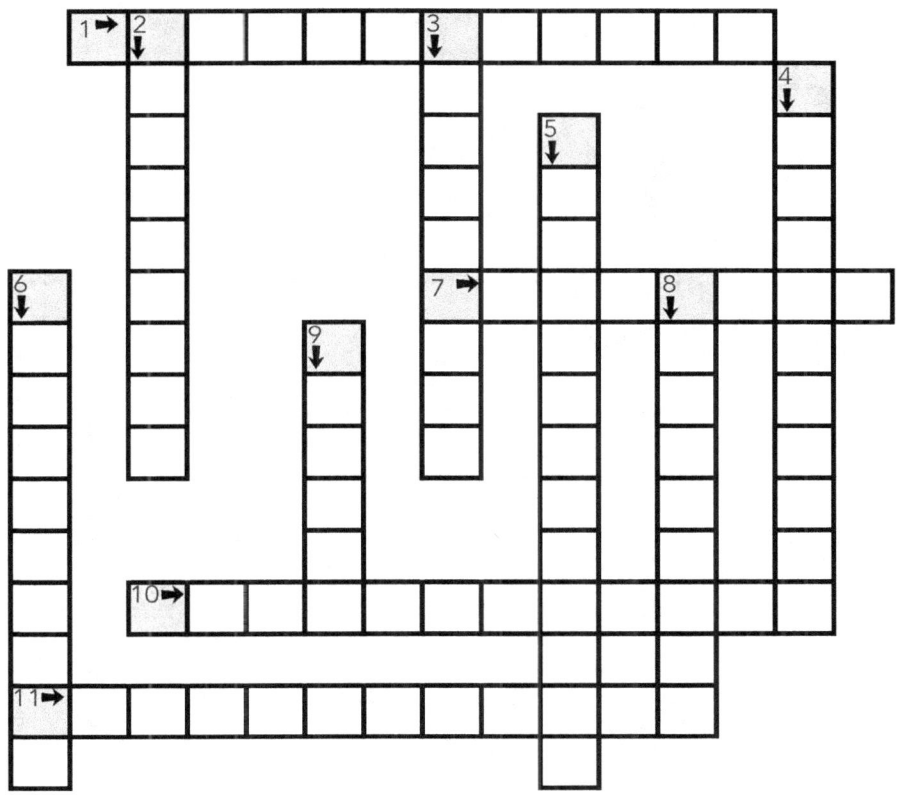

ACROSS

1. Novel cancer immunotherapy approach using messenger RNA technology.
7. Extracellular vesicles involved in intercellular communication and metastasis.
10. Combined diagnostic and therapeutic approach for personalized cancer treatment.
11. Study of metabolic profiles to identify cancer biomarkers.

DOWN

2. Computational analysis of medical images for cancer characterization.
3. Engineered T cells targeting specific cancer antigens.
4. Study of heritable changes in gene expression without DNA alteration.
5. Treatment approach based on genetic mutations rather than cancer type.
6. Role of gut bacteria in cancer development and immunotherapy response.
8. Three-dimensional tissue cultures mimicking tumor microenvironments for research.
9. Gene-editing tool for precise cancer cell modification studies.

Solution on page 107

PUZZLE 87
SMART IMPLANTS

Medical innovations and breakthroughs

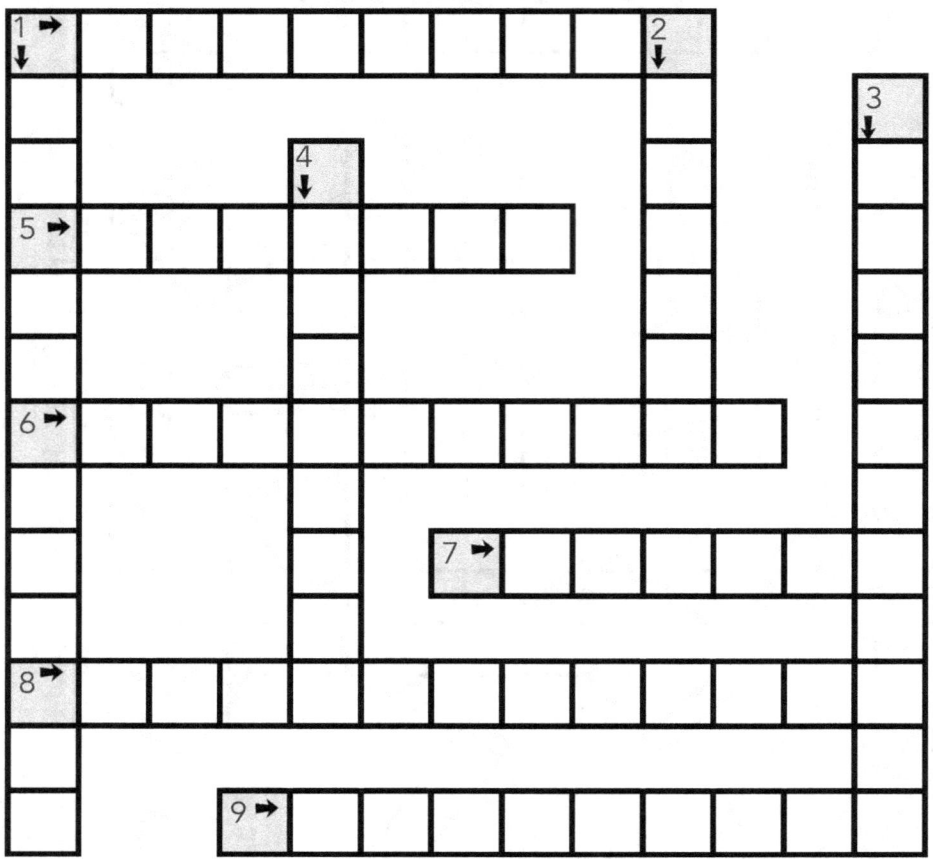

ACROSS

1. Implantable device tracking physiological parameters in real-time.
5. Inner ear implant restoring auditory function in hearing-impaired patients.
6. Field developing artificial limbs and body parts for amputees.
7. Miniature detectors in smart implants measuring various biological signals.
8. Material gradually absorbed by body after serving medical purpose.
9. Artificial replacement for missing body part or organ.

DOWN

1. Material harmoniously coexisting with living tissue without adverse effects.
2. Relating to computer-controlled mechanical devices in medical implants.
3. Integration of biological and electronic components in medical devices.
4. Conductive component in implants for electrical stimulation or recording.

Solution on page 107

PUZZLE 88
CRISPR GENE EDITING

Medical innovations and breakthroughs

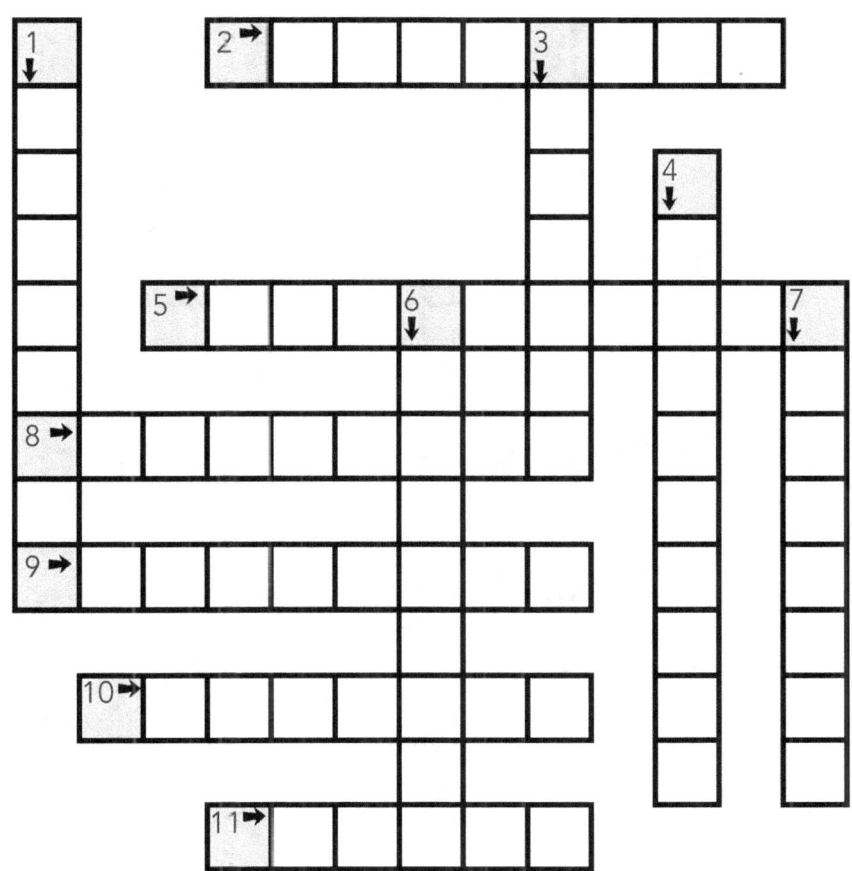

ACROSS

2. Genetic variation among cells within single organism.
5. Precise DNA modification without double-strand breaks.
8. Technique to alter inheritance in population.
9. Genetic material transferred between unrelated organisms.
10. Inactivation of specific gene to study function.
11. Programmable nucleases for targeted genome editing.

DOWN

1. Unintended genetic modifications in CRISPR editing.
3. A crucial enzyme used in CRISPR to cut DNA strands.
4. Modified using CRISPR gene editing technology.
6. Heritable chemical modifications affecting gene expression.
7. RNA sequence directing Cas9 to target DNA.

Solution on page 107

PUZZLE 89
DEFENDERS AGAINST VIRUSES

Medical innovations and breakthroughs

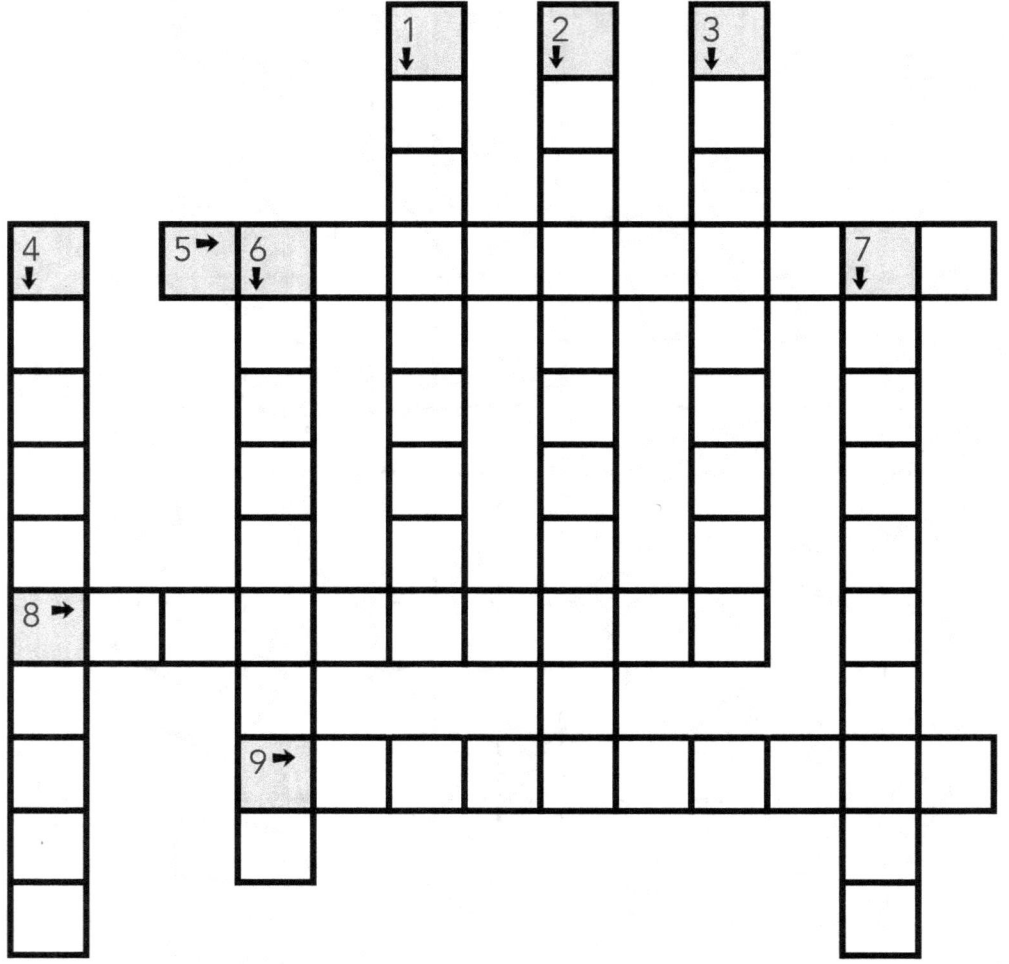

ACROSS

5. NS3/4A protease inhibitor for hepatitis C virus treatment.
8. Novel nucleoside reverse transcriptase translocation inhibitor for HIV.
9. Cytokine with antiviral properties used in hepatitis therapy.

DOWN

1. Guanosine analog antiviral drug for herpes virus infections.
2. NS5A inhibitor component in combination hepatitis C treatments.
3. Nucleoside analog reverse transcriptase inhibitor for hepatitis B.
4. Non-nucleoside reverse transcriptase inhibitor for HIV treatment.
6. Protease inhibitor used in combination antiretroviral HIV therapy.
7. Molecules that block specific viral replication processes.

Solution on page 107

PUZZLE 90
BIOLOGICS : THE NEXT GENERATION OF MEDICINE

Medical innovations and breakthroughs

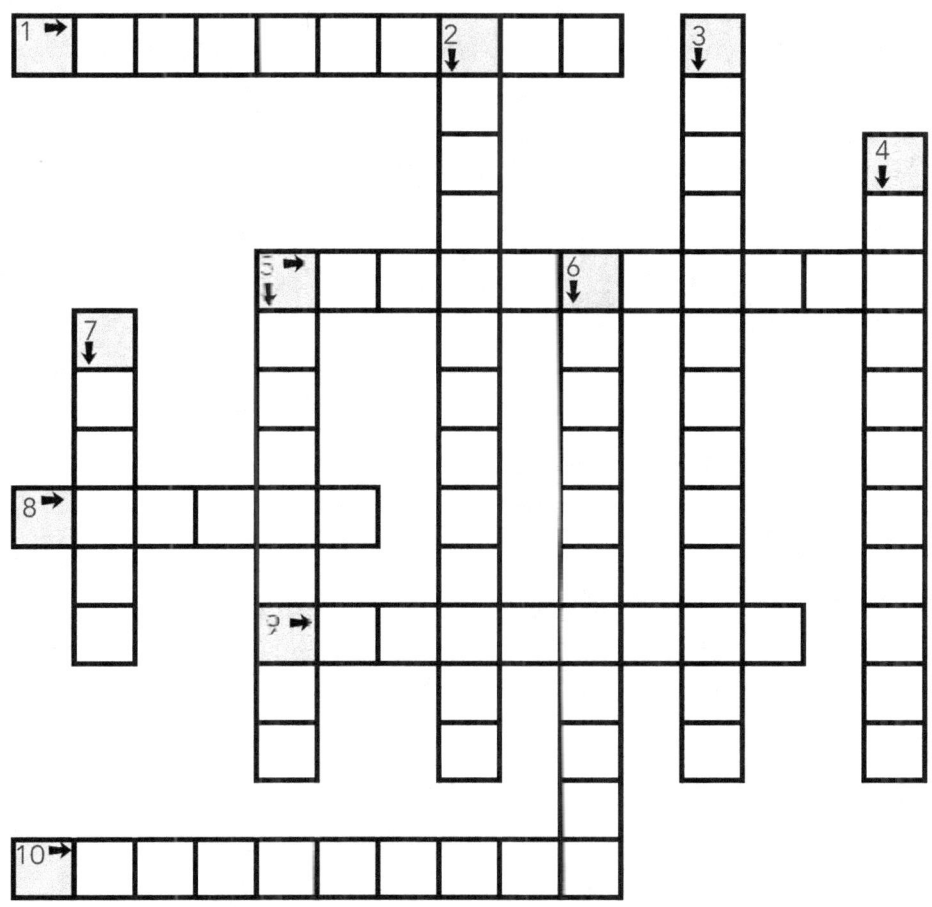

ACROSS

1. Monoclonal antibody targeting tumor necrosis factor alpha.
5. DNA technology used to produce therapeutic proteins.
8. Molecule that binds to specific receptor proteins.
9. Anti-CD20 antibody used in lymphoma treatment.
10. Large-scale study of protein structure and function.

DOWN

2. Large complex molecule like proteins or nucleic acids.
3. Treatment harnessing immune system to fight disease.
4. Cytokine involved in immune system cell signaling.
5. Biotechnology company pioneering antibody-based therapies.
6. Highly similar versions of existing biologic drugs.
7. Adalimumab, used to treat autoimmune disorders.

Solution on page 107

SOLUTIONS

PUZZLE 1:

ACROSS: 1. Beta-blocker, 4. Coronary, 5. Stress test, 7. Catheter, 8. Arrhythmia, 10. Pericardium, 11. Infarction.

DOWN: 1. Bypass, 2. Myocardium, 3. Atrium, 6. Stent, 8. Aorta, 9. Heart.

PUZZLE 2:

ACROSS: 1. CT scan, 4. Migraine, 7. Dendrite, 8. Meningitis, 9. Axon, 10. Tremor, 11. Synapse.

DOWN: 2. Stroke, 3. Thalamus, 4. Myelin, 5. Neuron, 6. Vertigo, 7. Dementia.

PUZZLE 3:

ACROSS: 1. Bone marrow, 8. Oncogene, 9. Remission, 10. Sarcoma, 11. Tumor.

DOWN: 2. Angiogenesis, 3. Malignant, 4. PET scan, 5. Leukemia, 6. Oncologist, 7. Carcinoma.

PUZZLE 4:

ACROSS: 2. Melanoma, 4. Cellulitis, 9. Epidermis, 10. Psoriasis.

DOWN: 1. Folliculitis, 3. Acne vulgaris, 4. Cryotherapy, 5. UV therapy, 6. Eczema, 7. Biopsy, 8. Patch test.

PUZZLE 5:

ACROSS: 4. Bone density, 5. Humerus, 7. X-ray, 9. Ligament, 11. Synovial fluid, 12. Scoliosis, 13. Splint.

DOWN: 1. Osteoblast, 2. Femur, 3. CT scan, 6. Ulna, 8. Meniscus, 10. Tibia.

PUZZLE 6:

ACROSS: 2. Colon, 6. Dyspepsia, 9. Hepatitis, 10. IBS, 11. Rectum, 12. Biopsy.

DOWN: 1. Endoscopy, 3. Appendicitis, 4. H pylori, 5. Liver, 7. Cirrhosis, 8. Jaundice.

PUZZLE 7:

ACROSS: 3. Bronchi, 5. Sleep apnea, 6. Hemoptysis, 7. Pulmonologist, 9. Inhaler, 10. Sputum, 11. Asthma.

DOWN: 1. Wheezing, 2. Ventilator, 4. Alveoli, 7. Pleura, 8. Lungs.

PUZZLE 8:

ACROSS: 2. Glucagon, 6. Pituitary, 9. Insulin, 10. Diabetes, 11. Graves' disease.

DOWN: 1. Prolactin, 3. Leptin, 4. Goiter, 5. Hypothalamus, 7. Thyroiditis, 8. Aldosterone.

PUZZLE 9:

ACROSS: 1. Biopsy, 3. Hemodialysis, 6. Kidney, 8. Renal, 10. Edema, 11. Tubules, 12. Uremia.

DOWN: 2. Podocytes, 4. Diuretic, 5. Hematuria, 7. Nephron, 9. Azotemia.

PUZZLE 10:

ACROSS: 1. Arthritis, 3. Rheumatoid, 5. Inflammation, 7. C-reactive, 8. Lupus, 10. Psoriatic, 11. Erythrocyte.

DOWN: 1. Autoimmune, 2. Biologics, 4. Anti-CCP, 6. Flare-up, 9. Gout.

PUZZLE 11:

ACROSS: 2. LASIK, 4. Dry eye, 5. Pupil, 9. Amblyopia, 12. Cornea, 13. Uveitis, 14. Cataract.

DOWN: 1. Retina, 2. Lens, 3. Sclera, 6. Vitreous, 7. Optic nerve, 8. Hyperopia, 10. Myopia, 11. Iris.

PUZZLE 12:

ACROSS: 1. Sinusitis, 5. Cerumen, 9. Dysphonia, 10. Vertigo, 11. Epistaxis.

DOWN: 2. Uvula, 3. Tinnitus, 4. Anosmia, 5. Cochlea, 6. Nasopharynx, 7. Laryngitis, 8. Otoscope.

PUZZLE 13:

ACROSS: 1. Erythrocytes, 5. Plasma, 9. Platelets, 10. Anemia, 11. Hemostasis

DOWN: 2. Thalassemia, 3. Hemophilia, 4. Leukemia, 6. Heparin, 7. Stem cells, 8. Hemolysis.

PUZZLE 14:

ACROSS: 4. Diaper rash, 6. Swaddling, 8. Growth chart, 10. Pacifier.

DOWN: 1. Measles, 2. Bronchiolitis, 3. Asthma inhaler, 5. Teething, 7. Apgar score, 9. Otoscope.

PUZZLE 15:

ACROSS: 2. Hospice, 5. Medicare, 6. Dementia, 7. Aging, 8. Frailty, 9. Elderly, 10. Sarcopenia.

DOWN: 1. Polypharmacy, 3. Incontinence, 4. Hearing loss.

PUZZLE 16:

ACROSS: 1. Ultrasound, 4. C-section, 6. Folic acid, 9. Epidural, 10. Uterus, 11. Episiotomy.
DOWN: 2. Amniocentesis, 3. Menopause, 5. Pregnancy, 7. Cervix, 8. Doula.

PUZZLE 17:

ACROSS: 2. Freud, 6. Adler, 7. Jung, 9. Beck, 10. Erikson, 11. Antipsychotic.
DOWN: 1. Anxiolytic, 3. Depression, 4. Agoraphobia, 5. Mindfulness, 8. Maslow.

PUZZLE 18:

ACROSS: 1. Bone density, 8. Mammogram, 9. PET scan, 10. SPECT, 11. Radioactive.
DOWN: 2. Sonogram, 3. Thyroid uptake, 4. Radiopaque, 5. Tomography, 6. Roentgen, 7. Gamma camera.

PUZZLE 19:

ACROSS: 1. Propofol, 4. Midazolam, 6. Ketamine, 9. Sedation, 10. Isoflurane, 11. Desflurane.
DOWN: 2. Remifentanil, 3. Lidocaine, 5. Fentanyl, 7. Epidural, 8. Opioid.

PUZZLE 20:

ACROSS: 2. Incontinence, 6. Nephrectomy, 8. Nocturia, 10. Prostate, 11. Creatinine.
DOWN: 1. Diuretic, 3. Nephron, 4. Urodynamics, 5. Hematuria, 7. Kidney, 9. Ureter.

PUZZLE 21:

ACROSS: 4. Antimicrobial, 8. Outbreak, 9. Transmission, 10. Vector-borne, 11. Nosocomial.
DOWN: 1. Pandemic, 2. PCR test, 3. ELISA, 5. Incubation, 6. Airborne, 7. Zoonotic.

PUZZLE 22:

ACROSS: 5. NK cells, 6. Antigens, 8. Adjuvants, 10. Epitopes, 11. Allergy.
DOWN: 1. Herd immunity, 2. Vaccines, 3. Antibodies, 4. Allergens, 7. Spleen, 9. T cells.

PUZZLE 23:

ACROSS: 2. Hematoxylin, 4. Microscope, 5. Sarcoma, 8. Autopsy, 10. Frozen section, 11. Lesion, 12. Benign.
DOWN: 1. Biopsy, 3. Microtome, 6. Apoptosis, 7. Histology, 9. Eosin.

PUZZLE 24:

ACROSS: **1.** Dermabrasion, **5.** Cleft palate, **9.** Chemical peels, **10.** Otoplasty, **11.** Scalpel.

DOWN: **2.** Botox, **3.** Silicone, **4.** Liposuction, **6.** Tummy tuck, **7.** Collagen, **8.** Nose job.

PUZZLE 25:

ACROSS: **3.** Code blue, **7.** Stroke, **9.** Ventilator, **10.** Trauma, **11.** Laryngoscope.

DOWN: **1.** Sepsis, **2.** Overdose, **4.** Defibrillator, **5.** EpiPen, **6.** Chest pain, **8.** Shock.

PUZZLE 26:

ACROSS: **1.** Cell division, **4.** Hepatitis C, **6.** Stem cells, **9.** Telomeres, **10.** Gene editing.

DOWN: **2.** DNA structure, **3.** Insulin, **5.** Oncogenes, **7.** Malaria, **8.** Pasteur.

PUZZLE 27:

ACROSS: **1.** X-rays, **4.** Pasteur, **8.** Stem cells, **10.** Lister, **11.** Microscope, **12.** Salk.

DOWN: **2.** Antiseptic, **3.** Tuberculosis, **5.** Antibiotics, **6.** Insulin, **7.** Barnard, **9.** Aspirin

PUZZLE 28:

ACROSS: **1.** Yin and yang, **6.** Theurgy, **8.** Amulets, **9.** Ebers Papyrus, **10.** Asklepios, **11.** Meridians.

DOWN: **2.** Ayurveda, **3.** Galen, **4.** Apothecary, **5.** Moxibustion, **7.** Humoralism.

PUZZLE 29:

ACROSS: **7.** Smallpox, **10.** Louis Pasteur, **11.** Insulin.

DOWN: **1.** Anesthesia, **2.** Edward Jenner, **3.** Lobotomy, **4.** William Morton, **5.** Hippocrates, **6.** Stethoscope, **8.** Germ theory, **9.** Blood types.

PUZZLE 30:

ACROSS: **1.** Muscle mass, **3.** Andropause, **5.** Six-pack abs, **6.** Depression, **7.** Prostate exam, **8.** Testosterone, **9.** Sleep apnea.

DOWN: **1.** Midlife crisis, **2.** Vasectomy, **4.** PSA test.

PUZZLE 31:

ACROSS: **1.** Stethoscope, **3.** Heart monitor, **5.** Pacemaker, **6.** Pulse oximeter, **8.** X-ray, **9.** Ventilator, **10.** Wheelchairs.

DOWN: 1. Scalpel, 2. Catheter, 4. Hearing aid, 7. Syringe.

PUZZLE 32:

ACROSS: 1. Colonoscopy, 4. Scalpel, 5. Retractor, 6. Epidural, 8. Angioplasty, 9. Microsurgery, 10. Biopsy.

DOWN: 1. Cauterization, 2. Laser surgery, 3. Forceps, 7. Sutures.

PUZZLE 33:

ACROSS: 1. Diaphragm, 4. Bone marrow, 8. Circulatory, 9. Intestines, 10. Vertebrae, 11. Skeleton.

DOWN: 2. Aorta, 3. Epidermis, 5. Endocrine, 6. Biceps, 7. Cartilage.

PUZZLE 34:

ACROSS: 4. Mercury, 7. Sanitation, 8. E coli, 9. Asbestos, 10. Smog.

DOWN: 1. Lead poisoning, 2. Pesticides, 3. Food safety, 5. Carcinogens, 6. Rachel Carson.

PUZZLE 35:

ACROSS: 6. Fortified, 7. Fiber, 8. Meal prep, 9. Food label, 10. Ketogenic.

DOWN: 1. Protein, 2. Mediterranean, 3. Leafy greens, 4. Diabetes, 5. Minerals.

PUZZLE 36:

ACROSS: 2. Marie Stopes, 4. Perimenopause, 5. Menstruation, 6. Pregnancy, 7. Mammogram, 8. HPV vaccine, 9. Birth control.

DOWN: 1. Pap smear, 3. Ovarian cancer.

PUZZLE 37:

ACROSS: 1. Kinesiology, 4. Homeopathy, 6. Chakras, 7. Bach flowers, 8. Biofeedback, 9. Yoga therapy.

DOWN: 2. Energy healing, 3. Meridians, 4. Holistic, 5. Ayurveda.

PUZZLE 38:

ACROSS: 1. Giardiasis, 4. Oocyst, 7. Trophozoite, 9. Nematode, 10. Cestode, 11. Parasitemia.

DOWN: 2. Sporozoite, 3. Entamoeba, 5. Trichinella, 6. Zoonosis, 8. Trematode.

PUZZLE 39:

ACROSS: 1. Teratogen, 7. Venomous, 8. Xenobiotic, 9. Poison, 10. Toxin, 11. Antidote.

DOWN: 2. Ecotoxicology, 3. Dose-response, 4. Genotoxicity, 5. Carcinogen, 6. Chelation.

PUZZLE 40:

ACROSS: 2. Allosteric, 5. Helicase, 7. Nucleotides, 9. Coenzymes, 10. Amino acids, 11. Active site.

DOWN: 1. NADH, 3. Ribosomes, 4. Glycolysis, 6. Krebs cycle, 8. Ligase.

PUZZLE 41:

ACROSS: 4. Allocation, 6. Triage, 7. Beneficence, 8. Gene editing, 9. Justice.

DOWN: 1. Placebo effect, 2. Bioethics, 3. DNR order, 4. Autonomy, 5. Living will.

PUZZLE 42:

ACROSS: 1. Off-label use, 6. Polypharmacy, 7. Half-life, 9. Prodrug, 10. Antagonist, 11. Tylenol.

DOWN: 2. Beta-blocker, 3. Atorvastatin, 4. Pharmacophore, 5. Dose-response, 8. Drug-drug.

PUZZLE 43:

ACROSS: 1. Microscopy, 4. Salmonella, 6. Pneumonia, 7. Tuberculosis, 9. Probiotics, 10. Antibiogram, 11. Gram staining.

DOWN: 2. Culture, 3. Pili, 5. Plasmid, 8. Biofilm.

PUZZLE 44:

ACROSS: 2. Inotrope, 5. Dopamine, 7. IV fluids, 10. Narcan, 11. Ketamine.

DOWN: 1. Morphine, 3. Intubation, 4. Adenosine, 6. Atropine, 8. Fentanyl, 9. Diuretic.

PUZZLE 45:

ACROSS: 2. Fleming, 5. Spore, 8. Contamination, 9. Amanita, 10. Mycelium.

DOWN: 1. Microscopy, 2. Fruiting body, 3. Hyphae, 4. Candidiasis, 5. Sporangium, 6. Fungicide, 7. Linnaeus.

PUZZLE 46:

ACROSS: 1. Leukemia, 5. Triglycerides, 8. Hepatitis, 9. Ferritin, 10. Pap smear, 11. Tuberculosis, 12. Blood type.

DOWN: 2. Urinalysis, 3. Anemia, 4. Creatinine, 6. Cholesterol, 7. Microscope.

PUZZLE 47:

ACROSS: 1. Fever, 3. Croup, 4. Leukemia, 5. Vaccination, 7. Measles, 10. Growth chart, 12. ADHD.

DOWN: 1. Food allergy, 2. Eczema, 3. Colic, 6. Teething, 8. Asthma, 9. Autism, 11. Rash.

PUZZLE 48:

ACROSS: 1. Pandemic, 3. Lysis, 4. Lwoff, 5. ELISA, 7. Virion, 8. Remdesivir, 9. Zoonosis.

DOWN: 1. Pasteur, 2. Ebola, 6. Rabies, 7. Virus.

PUZZLE 49:

ACROSS: 2. Lyme disease, 6. Tularemia, 7. Epidemic, 10. Tropical, 11. Chikungunya.

DOWN: 1. Fleas, 3. Malaria, 4. Eradication, 5. Repellent, 8. Plague, 9. Ebola.

PUZZLE 50:

ACROSS: 5. BMJ, 7. H Index, 9. Open Access, 11. The MJA, 12. The Lancet.

DOWN: 1. Wellcome Open, 2. PubMed Central, 3. NEJM, 4. Fauci, 6. Neurology, 8. JAMA, 10. Cell.

PUZZLE 51 (Diabetes Mellitus) :

ACROSS: 4. Insulin, 6. Beta cells, 9. Pancreas, 10. Polyuria, 11. Hyperglycemia, 12. Glucose.

DOWN: 1. Carbohydrates, 2. Nephropathy, 3. Metformin, 5. Sulfonylureas, 7. Gestational, 8. Neuropathy.

PUZZLE 52 (Hypertension)):

ACROSS: 2. Heart attack, 4. Diuretics, 8. Proteinuria, 9. Renin, 10. DASH Diet.

DOWN: 1. Retinopathy, 3. Aldosterone, 5. Systolic, 6. Stroke risk, 7. Diastolic.

PUZZLE 53(Asthma):

ACROSS: 2. Albuterol, 4. Rescue inhaler, 5. Inhalers, 7. Pet dander, 8. Leukotriene, 9. Montelukast.

DOWN: 1. Spirometry, 3. Oral steroids, 6. Spacer, 7. Pollen.

PUZZLE 54 Chronic Obstructive Pulmonary Disease (COPD):

ACROSS: 2. Chest X-ray, 4. Tiotropium, 8. Dyspnea, 9. Oxygen therapy.

DOWN: 1. Smoking, 2. Cor pulmonale, 3. Emphysema, 5. Spirometry, 6. Pneumonia, 7. Nebulizer, 8. DLCO.

PUZZLE 55 Coronary Artery Disease (CAD):

ACROSS: 1. Bypass surgery, 3. Angioplasty, 8. Stenosis, 9. NSTEMI, 10. Stent.

DOWN: 1. Beta-blockers, 2. Placue, 4. Ischemia, 5. Stress test, 6. Troponin, 7. Aspirin, 8. Statins.

PUZZLE 56 (Stroke):

ACROSS: 1. Dysarthria, 3. Thrombotic, 5. CT angiogram, 6. Aphasia, 8. Dysphagia, 9. Embolic.

DOWN: 1. Door-to-needle, 2. Hemiparesis, 4. Broca's area, 7. Ataxia.

PUZZLE 57 (Rheumatoid Arthritis):

ACROSS: 5. Bone erosion, 6. Synovitis, 7. Inflammation, 9. Methotrexate, 1. Flare-up, 12. Remission.

DOWN: 1. Cartilage, 2. Pannus, 3. Deformity, 4. Autoimmune, 8. Fatigue, 10. X-rays.

PUZZLE 58 (Chronic Kidney Disease):

ACROSS: 1. Acidosis, 4. Edema, 7. Azotemia, 8. Dialysis, 9. Glomerular, 10. Filtration.

DOWN: 1. Anemia, 2. Diuretics, 3. Nephrologist, 5. Uremia, 6. Parathyroid.

PUZZLE 59 (Osteoporosis):

ACROSS: 1. Density, 3. Genetics, 6. Estrogen, 7. Medication, 9. Collagen, 10. Nutrition, 11. Fosamax.

DOWN: 1. Denosumab, 2. Screening, 4. Smoking, 5. Vitamin D, 8. Calcium.

PUZZLE 60 (Alzheimer's Disease):

ACROSS: 4. Amyloid, 5. Apraxia, 8. Memantine, 9. Agitation, 10. Aricept.

DOWN: 1. Delusions, 2. Rivastigmine, 3. Galantamine, 6. Namenda, 7. Dementia.

PUZZLE 61 (Parkinson's Disease):

ACROSS: 1. Motor cortex, 4. Cognitive, 5. L-dopa, 8. Freezing, 9. Posture, 10. Gait, 11. Tremors.

DOWN: 1. Micrographia, 2. Trembling, 3. Balance, 6. Rigidity, 7. Neural, 8. Fatigue.

PUZZLE 62 (Peptic Ulcer Disease):

ACROSS: 1. Dyspepsia, 4. Bleeding, 7. Mucosa, 9. Proton, 10. Endoscopy.

DOWN: 1. Duodenum, 2. Acidic, 3. Perforation, 4. Bloating, 5. Epigastric, 6. Gastritis, 8. Biopsy.

PUZZLE 63 Irritable Bowel Syndrome (IBS):

ACROSS: 1. Probiotics, 3. Flatulence, 6. Diarrhea, 7. Motility, 8. Constipation, 9. Gluten-free, 10. Loperamide, 11. Colonoscopy.

DOWN: 1. Peppermint oil, 2. Dietary fiber, 4. Abdominal pain, 5. Bloating.

PUZZLE 64 (Hepatitis):

ACROSS: 1. Cholestasis, 2. Transaminase, 5. Cirrhosis, 7. Bilirubin, 8. Viremia, 9. Interferon, 10. Splenomegaly.

DOWN: 1. Cytokines, 3. Ascites, 4. Jaundice, 6. Ribavirin.

PUZZLE 65 (HIV AIDS):

ACROSS: 1. Receptor, 4. Replication, 8. Opportunistic, 9. Nevirapine, 10. Adherence.

DOWN: 2. Cytokine, 3. Protease, 4. Retrovirus, 5. Seroconvert, 6. Kaposi, 7. Ritonavir.

PUZZLE 66 (Tuberculosis):

ACROSS: 1. Isoniazid, 5. Droplets, 6. Rifampin, 7. Isolation, 9. Sputum, 10. Granuloma, 11. Cavitary.

DOWN: 2. Dyspnea, 3. Bacilli, 4. Coughing, 5. Dormancy, 8. Latency.

PUZZLE 67 (Anemia):

ACROSS: 1. Aplastic, 6. Dyspnea, 7. Megaloblastic, 8. Transfusion, 10. Pallor, 11. Chelation.

DOWN: 2. Cobalamin, 3. Ferritin, 4. Microcytic, 5. Hematocrit, 9. Folate.

PUZZLE 68 (Thyroid Disorders):

ACROSS: 1. Pretibial, 7. Synthroid, 8. Radioiodine, 9. Antithyroid.

DOWN: 1. Palpitations, 2. Bradycardia, 3. Thyroiditis, 4. Myxedema, 5. Tachycardia, 6. Euthyroid.

PUZZLE 69 (Depression and Anxiety):

ACROSS: 1. Dysthymia, 7. Obsessive, 9. Despair, 11. Counseling, 12. Serotonin, 13. Melancholy.

DOWN: 2. Self-esteem, 3. Anhedonia, 4. Restlessness, 5. Mindfulness, 6. Isolation, 8. Irritability, 10. Insomnia.

PUZZLE 70 Dermatitis (eczema):

ACROSS: 1. Pustules, 4. Patch, 6. Pruritus, 7. Atopy, 9. Plaques, 11. Vesicles, 12. Allergen, 13. Crusting.

DOWN: 2. Excoriation, 3. Xerosis, 5. Erythema, 8. Papules, 10. Edema.

PUZZLE 71 Venous Thromboembolism (VTE):

ACROSS: 1. Tachypnea, 5. Syncope, 8. Edema, 9. Orthopnea, 10. Dyspnea.

DOWN: 2. Palpitations, 3. Hypotension, 4. Tachycardia, 6. Cyanosis, 7. Hypoxia, 8. Erythema.

PUZZLE 72 (Leukemia):

ACROSS: 1. Neutropenia, 6. Fever, 9. Bruising, 10. Anemia.

DOWN: 2. Pallor, 3. Petechiae, 4. Fatigue, 5. Weight loss, 7. Epistaxis, 8. Bone pain, 9. Bleeding.

PUZZLE 73 (Meningitis):

ACROSS: 2. Confusion, 6. Brudzinski, 8. Diplopia, 10. Fever, 12. Tachycardia, 13. Vomiting, 14. Papilledema.

DOWN: 1. Kernig, 3. Seizures, 4. Nuchal rigidity, 5. Photophobia, 7. Delirium, 9. Petechiae, 11. Myalgia.

PUZZLE 74 (Endometriosis):

ACROSS: 1. Infertility, 4. Endometrial, 7. Nodules, 9. Dysmenorrhea, 12. Fibrosis.

DOWN: 2. Tenderness, 3. Ovarian, 5. Menorrhagia, 6. Rectal, 8. Dyspareunia, 9. Dysuria, 10. Fatigue, 11. Biopsy.

PUZZLE 75 (Polycythemia Vera):

ACROSS: 1. Hyperuricemia, 3. Hypertension, 5. Thrombosis, 9. Tinnitus, 10. Gout, 11. Dyspnea.

DOWN: 1. Hepatomegaly, 2. Paresthesia, 3. Hemorrhage, 4. Epistaxis, 6. Plethora, 7. Cyanosis, 8. Vertigo.

PUZZLE 76:

ACROSS: 5. Phage, 9. Resensitize, 10. Superbugs.

DOWN: 1. Nanoparticles, 2. Polymyxins, 3. Bacteriocins, 4. Metagenomics, 6. Ribosome, 7. Halicin, 8. CRISPR.

PUZZLE 77:

<u>ACROSS:</u> **1.** Sequencing, **2.** Genome mapping, **4.** Gene therapy, **5.** Stem cells, **8.** Nucleotides, **9.** Alleles, **10.** Hereditary, **11.** Epigenetics.

<u>DOWN:</u> **1.** Somatic cells, **3.** Genotype, **6.** Base pairs, **7.** Phenotype.

PUZZLE 78:

<u>ACROSS:</u> **1.** Scalpel, **6.** Aseptic, **8.** Retractor, **9.** Endoscopy.

<u>DOWN:</u> **1.** Sterilization, **2.** Lister, **3.** Chloroform, **4.** Kocher, **5.** Laparotomy, **6.** Autoclave, **7.** Halsted.

PUZZLE 79:

<u>ACROSS:</u> **1.** Leadless, **5.** Electrode, **8.** Telemetry, **9.** Photovoltaic.

<u>DOWN:</u> **2.** Electrophysiology, **3.** Defibrillator, **4.** Implantation, **6.** Repolarization, **7.** Synchronization.

PUZZLE 80:

<u>ACROSS:</u> **1.** Scattering, **7.** Synchrotron, **9.** Mammogram, **10.** Fluoroscopy.

<u>DOWN:</u> **2.** Attenuation, **3.** Angiogram, **4.** Dosimetry, **5.** Penumbra, **6.** Collimator, **8.** Radiomics.

PUZZLE 81:

<u>ACROSS:</u> **1.** Bexsero, **5.** Pandemic, **9.** Immunization, **11.** Ervebo.

<u>DOWN:</u> **2.** RSVpreF, **3.** Chikungunya, **4.** Dengvaxia, **6.** NSCLC, **7.** Hecolin, **8.** Tetanus, **10.** ZPIV.

PUZZLE 82:

<u>ACROSS:</u> **4.** Validation, **6.** Processing, **7.** Cohort, **8.** Biomarker, **9.** Predictive, **11.** Modeling.

<u>DOWN:</u> **1.** Accuracy, **2.** Algorithm, **3.** Mining, **5.** Deep Learning, **10.** EHR.

PUZZLE 83:

<u>ACROSS:</u> **1.** Reconstructive, **3.** Stem Cells, **6.** Chimeric, **8.** Osteoblast, **9.** Scaffolding, **10.** Bioprinting, **11.** Functionalization.

<u>DOWN:</u> **2.** Tissue Engineering, **4.** Autologous, **5.** Cell Therapy, **7.** Reprogramming.

PUZZLE 84:

ACROSS: 5. Intraoperative, 6. Sutureless, 7. Transcatheter, 8. Cryosurgery, 9. Endoscopy.

DOWN: 1. Robotics, 2. Biomaterials, 3. Tele-surgery, 4. Smart Sutures.

PUZZLE 85:

ACROSS: 1. MRNA vaccines, 7. Exosomes, 10. Theranostics, 11. Metabolomics.

DOWN: 2. Radiomics, 3. CAR-T cells, 4. Epigenetics, 5. Tumor-agnostic, 6. Microbiome, 8. Organoids, 9. CRISPR.

PUZZLE 86:

ACROSS: 2. Peptide-based, 4. Viral vectors, 5. CNS delivery, 8. RNA-based drugs, 9. Microbubbles, 10. Gene therapy, 11. Transcranial.

DOWN: 1. Nanocarrier, 3. Exosomes, 6. Liposomes, 7. Neurotech.

PUZZLE 87:

ACROSS: 1. Rhodiola, 3. BetaVia, 8. Non-GMO, 9. Elderberry, 10. Adaptogens.

DOWN: 1. Reishi, 2. DailyZz, 4. Ashwagandha, 5. Ginseng, 6. Nootropics, 7. Cordyceps.

PUZZLE 88:

ACROSS: 2. Mosaicism, 5. Base-editing, 8. Gene-drive, 9. Transgene, 10. Knockout, 11. TALENs.

DOWN: 1. Off-target, 3. Cas-nine, 4. Crisprized, 6. Epigenome, 7. Guide RNA.

PUZZLE 89:

ACROSS: 5. Glecaprevir, 8. Islatravir, 9. Interferon.

DOWN: 1. Acyclovir, 2. Velpatasvir, 3. Entecavir, 4. Doravirine, 6. Lopinavir, 7. Inhibitors.

PUZZLE 90:

ACROSS: 1. Infliximab, 5. Recombinant, 8. Ligand, 9. Rituximab, 10. Proteomics.

DOWN: 2. Macromolecule, 3. Immunotherapy, 4. Interleukin, 5. Regeneron, 6. Biosimilars, 7. Humira.

www.ingramcontent.com/pod-product-compliance
Lightning Source LLC
Chambersburg PA
CBHW062111220526
45471CB00010B/3696